Love Your Body

Your Path to Transformation, Health, and Healing

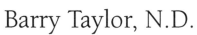

Barry Taylor, N.D.

Creator of the renowned "Love Your Body" program

with Luke Taylor

Contents

*I dedicate this book to my parents
for overcoming the struggles and suffering they endured
in their lives, and persevering to create a life and home
that has made me the man I am today.*

Author's Note

The names and circumstances detailed in the case histories shared in this book have been changed to protect the privacy of the individuals involved. In some instances, stories are shared as a composite to more clearly articulate the point at hand.

Acknowledgements

There are many people who have been instrumental in bringing this book to completion and to whom I owe my sincere thanks.

First to Nicole Buchman, Dr. Stephen Bochner, Jack Rothchild, Lee Weinstein, Dr. Peter Kevorkian, Evan Mulvaney, Joan and Steve Belkin, Jaclyn Bennett, Bill Twist, and Harry Peeples for reading the early drafts and offering their loving, heartfelt support. To Cheryl Stone for her invaluable editorial wisdom and copy editing. To Eileen Daily for her ongoing generous feedback and support. To Harv Ecker, Blair Singer, Larry Gilman, Adam Markel, and Joel Roberts for their encouragement, wisdom, and guidance. To the men of Primal Dog for holding me accountable to be the best person I can be. To Bill and Lynne Twist for generously allowing me to bring the writing of this book to completion in their home.

To my heroes and teachers who have shared their wisdom and love with me throughout my life: Virginia Fidel, Jeff Bland, Raz Ingrasci, Werner Erhard, David Deida, Alison Armstrong and Louis

Billotte. Your guidance and generosity have had an immeasurable impact on how I live in the world.

Finally, to my two sons, Jacob and Luke.

Jacob provided wonderful insight and feedback on the final draft of this book, for which I am very grateful. He is following his own path in medicine. Jacob recently received a master's of public health and is beginning medical school focusing on community health and integrative medicine.

Luke has been my full partner in creating this book as a labor of love. He has taken my ideas, organized them, re-articulated them, and expanded on them, giving them structure and cohesion. His coaching as a skilled writer and editor has been utterly invaluable. In addition to the joy of completing this, my first book, having my son as my partner throughout the process was an unforeseen and indescribable bonus.

Foreword

By Jeffrey Bland, Ph.D., FACN, FACB

First let me "come clean"—I have known Dr. Barry Taylor since 1976 when he was a student of mine during his last year in medical school at the National College of Naturopathic Medicine in Portland, Oregon. He has been my professional colleague and friend ever since.

With that said, I do think that I can provide an objective evaluation of his book, *Love Your Body: Your Path to Transformation, Health and Healing*. Dr. Taylor's approach to healing is more than just about diet, nutrition, lifestyle, or the body-mind experience. He is interested in holistic wellbeing, in its deepest sense, and the synergy between the mind, spirit, and body. I believe that Dr. Taylor has tuned, refined, and polished his practice over the past thirty plus years to be a standard of excellence from which other health and healing programs are evaluated. What I have always appreciated about Dr. Taylor is his commitment to making his programs focused on the patient experience, rather than any particular dogma or prescription. His approach is so effective because it can be understood and successfully applied by all types of people at different ages and states of health who are aspiring to gain higher function, for their bodies, emotional capacities, and psyche.

In 1978 I asked Dr. Taylor to be a guest lecturer in a course called "Is There a Healer in the House?" that I offered at the Evergreen State College in Olympia, Washington. Even at that early stage in his career, he was connecting the different dots that contribute to wellbeing, which to many seem separate and distinct. Many of the students in the class who heard Dr. Taylor's message became the first students at the Bastyr College of Naturopathic Medicine, which we founded in 1980. Since then, Dr. Taylor's Love Your Body Program has provided transformation for those who go through it because it is transformational in its conception and content; it has been Dr. Taylor's proving ground for nearly 40 years.

This book has the opportunity to help countless numbers of aspirants who are looking for an approach to recreating the good health they may have felt at a previous time in their lives, or for those looking to discover a more profound sense of health than they ever knew they could experience.

The wisdom in this book comes from decades of self-study, philosophical refinement, and real world experience in clinical practice that defines the past 36 years of Dr. Taylor's life history. It addresses in a very non-threatening way the difficult question we all face at one time or another: why aren't I happy with myself? It provides real tools for both self-evaluation and skill development in learning how to love yourself. It teaches the reader how to be in charge of their own life. It builds resilience, self-esteem, and improvement in vitality, while offering practical insight into the elements that contribute to or detract from our sense of wellness. Fundamentally, this book is empowering and fun to engage in, but, ultimately, it is an invitation to embody a more complete sense of wellness, peace, and love than you may have thought was possible.

It has been a wonderful experience for me to see how Dr. Taylor has used his gifts and talents to help so many over his years in practice, and to now make his approach to health and healing available to everyone through this marvelous book.

Jeffrey Bland, Ph.D., FACN, FACB
President, Personalized Lifestyle Medicine Institute
June 2013

The two most important days of your life are the
day you are born, and the day you find out why.

— Mark Twain

Introduction

Growing up, I was sick all the time. I had strep throat with 103-104 degree temperatures three to four times a year, for four consecutive years. I spent what felt like months on penicillin and antibiotics, headaches plagued me almost daily and I popped aspirin like candy (which I also had a taste for). During my freshman year of college, I was actually hospitalized for internal bleeding from all the aspirin I took. My body and I were not friends.

Then, in 1970 my college advisor introduced me to Dr. Louis Billotte who became one of the most influential people in my life. Dr. B, as many of his patients called him, was a miracle worker for the clients who came from all over the world to consult with him in his home just north of Boston. Receiving his M.D. in 1930 and his N.D. degree in 1932, he was one of those rare doctors who knew that the limits of extraordinary health and healing were well beyond what most people considered possible. As a young student I came to practically worship Dr. Billotte. He became my mentor and guide, and I had a standing appointment with him every Monday at 9 A.M., which I kept for years. In my first year of following his counsel, I took handfuls of vitamins, desiccated liver powder, cod liver oil, and nutritional yeast every day. He asked me to begin looking carefully at what I was eating, encouraging me to choose food that was grown organically and was minimally processed. I was also clocking nearly four hours of yoga daily and learning to make peace with my mind through meditation. The new good health I was experiencing under Dr. Billotte's care was a revelation and became the focus of my life.

In the second year of seeing Dr. Billotte, he asked me if I was ready for the next level. I trusted this man totally, and without hesitation began increasingly intensive periods of cleansing and detoxification. I fasted one day per week to rest my body. On Mondays, I drank only fresh vegetable juice and water. That lasted for a year, at which point Dr. B asked me to add two extra days of juice only in the fourth week of each month. In the third year, I added another two full weeks of cleansing at the end of each quarter, around the equinox and solstice. Some of those longer cleanses lasted three to six weeks at a time.

I felt incredible. By the time I went to naturopathic school, I was logging over 100 days of cleansing per year, and while I recognize that this was radical to some degree, it also gave me a treasure trove of experience to bring into my naturopathic medical school training.

Over the past nearly 40 years of practicing medicine in New England, I have worked with thousands of patients, supporting them in creating optimal health and a life rooted in transformational healing. Many of my clients come to me fed up with conventional medicine. When they go to see their physicians, their questions often go unanswered, their interactions can be brusque and impersonal, and, in too many cases, they don't get better. What I have found is that a fundamental understanding of what generates and sustains truly optimal health as well as what constitutes meaningful healing is absent, both in the mainstream medical establishment

HEALTH and HEALING

Health is a measure of complete physical, mental, emotional, and spiritual well-being. Healing is the process of restoring physical, mental, emotional, and spiritual wholeness. It is the experience of becoming connected to one's most essential spiritual nature and personal wholeness.

and in the public. Furthermore, doctors and patients often lack the ability to communicate with one another in a manner that empowers the healing process. This book is intended to help readers build a foundation of understanding from which optimal health and healing can naturally and continually flow into their lives.

From a holistic point of view, optimal health is not simply the absence of disease symptoms. Rather, it is a sense of being energetic, vital, and intentional about certain practices that result in ideal organ function and synergy, which create an enjoyable physical experience. When you know how to optimize your vital life systems, you have choices about how to increase your energy and stamina, how to strengthen your immune system, how to balance your hormones, how to lose and maintain weight, how to deal with stress and the demands of work, family, and your responsibilities all within a context of greater connection, peace, and wholeness.

Being sick and not feeling well is a challenge for a great many people. This book is especially for those who suffer from "vertical disease." Vertical disease is when you are not sick enough to be in bed, but have resigned yourself to chronic asthma, allergies, low energy, or coffee dependence; indigestion, bloating and distension plague you daily; your joints ache and arthritis is a constant distraction; you have recurrent headaches, continued susceptibility to infections, or your hormonal swings make certain times of the month seem out of control. If you are frustrated by your eating or other addictive patterns, if your weight is out of control and you are tired of dieting, this book will offer new tools and insights to help you get clear about the path forward. If you feel stressed, overwhelmed, tired, or your sex life is locked in the closet somewhere, this book is for you. And, if you are someone who gets sick often enough that you do have to be "horizontal," forcing you to miss work or putting a strain on your intimate relationships, this book is especially for you.

This book is laid out to provide a holistic understanding of the life-sustaining systems that support health and healing. It begins by looking at those individual physical systems within your body that maintain and contribute to optimal health. Then it looks at the context in which healing takes place and the different tools and practices you might consider using along your journey. When you finish reading this book, it is my intention that you will be excited about learning how to deepen your connection to healing and living from your empowered identity as someone who creates healing in your own life.

While we will discuss a number of concrete areas that affect health—including nutrition, the adrenal system, and the immune system—we will also look at your relationship to healing and the role you play in bringing healing more intentionally into your life. At the heart of a truly transformative healing context is the development and practice of awareness. For some, awareness is developed through certain meditation and mindfulness practices, while for others it might be writing and reflecting on your physical and emotional experience. Becoming a dispassionate observer of your physical, emotional, mental, and spiritual experiences—witnessing your experience without being swept up in any particular judgment or assessment—is vital to creating new possibilities for optimal health and healing in your life.

Health and Healing Tip:
What you Appreciate, Appreciates

Find or purchase a journal that you can dedicate to your healing process and title it "Healing in My Life." Over the course of the subsequent chapters, write your answers and reflections to these processes in this notebook and refer to them regularly to remind yourself of the insights and commitments that might arise.

Sit quietly for a few minutes and allow yourself to relax. Allow your breath to flow freely and naturally. Think of an image in your life that you consider beautiful. This might be a flower, a place you have visited that inspires you, the face of someone you love, or a work of art. Take the beauty of this image into your mind and heart. Breathe it in. Stay with this picture in your mind for at least a full minute and allow this experience of beauty to reach every cell of your body.

Now, on a clean sheet of paper in your journal write down everything you are grateful for about your physical body. Make a specific list of anything and everything you can acknowledge that works. How does your body help you experience this multi-dimensional world of colors, sounds, and sensations? Acknowledge how you depend on your body for the vast amount of what you experience in your life. Be specific.

When you are finished, re-read what you have written about the aspects of your body that you can acknowledge with a bow of respect and gratitude.

Note: Many of the visualizations and exercises offered throughout this book are best read and then undertaken. In some cases, it may be helpful to read the instructions well enough to understand them, then set the book aside and go through the practice.

As you read this book, it may also be useful to keep in mind some of the following questions, allowing them to percolate in your awareness and open up new ways of seeing things.

- What is optimal health for me?
- How do I encourage my health?
- How do I impair or block my health?
- What does healing mean to me?
- Am I aware of how I heal?
- How do I block healing in my life?
- What would I need to more powerfully allow for healing in my life?

As the sections conclude, I will offer a few visualization practices, which are intended to help the information integrate into your body in a more holistic way, not staying confined to the conceptual framework of the mind. Hold these practices lightly and with curiosity, and accept the invitation to greater wellness and wellbeing as deeply as you can.

Chapter One

Models of Health and Healing

My father, George, was living the good retired life in South Florida. He and my mother had a beautiful apartment on the water and a community of friends they socialized with regularly. Then, at 86, he was taken to the hospital four times in three months for chest pains, being released each time with medication. I got a call that he was again on his way to the ER for severe chest pain, but this time they would keep him overnight and perform an angioplasty in the morning. Angioplasty is a procedure that inserts a tube into one of the coronary arteries in order to let more blood flow. I got on a plane immediately so I could be with my father when he got out of surgery.

When I arrived, I met with the cardiologist who was taking care of my father. He was a warm, cordial, friendly man who had gone to Boston University for medical school, and he shared that his morning surgery schedule of 45 angioplasties was a light day for him. The headquarters where we met was like a massive flight deck on the Starship Enterprise from Star Trek with dozens of control panels and monitors each beeping a different sound, tracking his patients' vital signs.

After we spoke a bit about my father, I went up to the recovery ward. Although he was a little groggy, George was his usual funny self. He wasn't in pain, but he was starving since he hadn't eaten anything in 36 hours. Soon, a lunch cart arrived for the 45 people in the recovery ward, each of whom had received an angioplasty that morning. As the tray was put in front of my salivating father, I looked with dismay at the roast beef, macaroni salad, cheese, white roll, and key lime pie with ice cream they were serving for lunch. Here was a group of people who had just undergone heart surgery to support better circulation to their hearts, which weren't functioning correctly, and their first meal post-operation was comprised of red meat, sugar, dairy, and white flour.

While performing an angioplasty might sometimes be critical to alleviating chest pain due to a blocked blood flow, I was struck by the contrast between the intention of the surgical procedure and the symbolism of the meal. When I mentioned this to my father's cardiologist, he nodded his head sympathetically and said, "I completely agree that lifestyle and diet impact the progression and development of disease, but it honestly wasn't our focus in medical school."

The cardiologist's response was not surprising. While some medical doctors believe in complementary therapies, most do not know how to integrate them into their practice. At hospitals, it's even more difficult to make adjustments, since vastly complex and bureaucratic systems determine much about procedure and protocol. Many medical institutions are way behind on the current research; not only do they perpetuate antiquated practices, but many of their policies actually aggravate or contribute to the diseases and symptoms they seek to alleviate. After a procedure like angioplasty, George's body needed foods that were both easy to digest and packed with dense nutrition that would help his tissues heal quickly. A meal of red meat, sugar, dairy, and white flour was actually an enormous burden on his body, given the trauma to his tissues from surgery.

Many patients think their doctors know everything there is to know about health, when in fact most medical doctors are trained in a very specific—and sometimes limited—medical model that focuses on disease removal and symptom alleviation, which is very different from creating, sustaining, and serving optimal health.

When most of us visit our doctor, we generally go seeking relief from the symptoms that ail us. If you have eczema, you want relief from your itchy skin; if you have arthritis, all you want is for the ache to go away. Similarly, most physicians are trained primarily to remove their patients' pain. Often times, however, the information we get from our health care providers does little to inform our understanding of the cause and origin of our symptoms. Rather, we are given a drug, a treatment, or told to adjust our diet, with the implication being that our symptoms are of singular origin, not the result of an interrelated system. Make the pain go away, and the problem disappears too, we think.

This is not just about how doctor's approach medicine, but also about how you, as an agent in your own healthcare, expect to be treated and how you understand your capacity to generate health in your own life. Both doctors and patients alike carry around an unconscious set of expectations for how health and healing work and what their respective roles in that process should be. This book is intended to give you a very different set of questions about your own healing process and the kind of relationship you have with your health care providers. You want to be able to question yourself and your beliefs about healing, as well as intentionally seek out the kind of partnership you wish to receive from those physicians.

We in the West have been undergoing a quiet revolution in the accessibility and acceptability of integrative medicine. The phrase "alternative medicine" as a marginalized paradigm of thinking has all but disappeared, and complementary and alternative medicine (CAM) is now an industry that generates billions of dollars per year.

The implications of such an industry are certainly complicated, but what it indicates is a shift in the conversation, values, and belief systems of the population.

Increasingly, consumers believe that there is more to health than drugs and surgery, and we have begun to collectively demand greater information and power to choose how we pursue our health. Awareness of the importance of organic produce has skyrocketed; more of us than ever practice yoga regularly and integrate meditation and mindfulness into our daily lives; there are even some medical schools that now offer elective courses in acupuncture and residencies in integrative medicine. The revolution is by no means complete, but it is in full swing.

The most important part of this revolution is a new willingness to question our beliefs about how health and healing work. This is actually quite an enormous undertaking, as most of us regard ideas or beliefs outside our familiar framework as strange and even hostile. Nearly three decades ago, for instance, acupuncture had not yet reached the mainstream and was regarded by many with suspicion and skepticism. Now, acupuncture is widespread and the wisdom of this 6000-year-old tradition is respected by more mainstream physicians and consumers.

This book will continue to illuminate some of the presuppositions that many of us hold about how health and healing operate in our lives. It will offer a model for approaching your health that is fundamentally empowering and takes a uniquely integrated perspective on how your mind, body, emotions, and spirit influence and connect with one another. The intention is that you leave with a greater sense of your own personal capacity and power for generating healing even as the circumstances of your life continue to change and grow. Keep an open mind and an open heart while you read, and you will undoubtedly come away with a powerful new paradigm with which to live your life.

UNDERSTANDING THE ALLOPATHIC
PARADIGM OF MEDICINE

From the advertisements we see for pills and drugs to the advice we get from most physicians and the examples we see in our friends and family, we live in a world that believes pain should be cured by magic bullets—a drug, a vitamin, dieting, exercise, or any single thing we imbue with the power to get us out of pain and discomfort. Before we know it, we too are going through life, unconsciously assuming that the answer to our ailments comes in the form of a magic bullet, and that when the pain is gone the problem is gone as well. We do this in part because we see pain in our culture as an irritating distraction from the regularly scheduled programming of our lives.

Another way to understand pain is as a signal that carries important information about the state of our health. Imagine you were awakened suddenly in the middle of the night by a terrible alarm going off somewhere in your house. The noise is so piercing that you knock the alarm off the wall as soon as you find it, silencing the terrible sound before you go back to bed. On the one hand, you have the peace of mind of not having to deal with the irritating noise, but on the other hand, you have done nothing to locate the trigger for the alarm. There may still be a fire burning in a hidden corner of your house.

For the most part, however, most of us—doctors and patients alike—do not see pain as a messenger of information that invites a deeper inquiry into its origin and purpose; pain is simply seen as bad, something to get rid of. This approach to treating pain and illness is known to many as the allopathic paradigm of medicine and it is the go-to methodology that most physicians in the United States employ in their practice. It is also how many of us unconsciously assume healing works. The word "allopathy" comes from the Greek *allos*, meaning "other" or "different" and the word pathos, meaning "feeling" or "suffering." The primary interest of allopathy is to treat the disease or symptom, not the individual; it is to have you feel something other than what you currently feel, which in some cases makes sense, but is rarely sufficient for true healing or for sustaining good health.

The science of allopathy depends on numbers and statistics. Massive hours of clinical research go into studying huge numbers of people with common symptoms in order to derive a common cause or relationship between their symptoms and what then gets categorized as an illness or disease. The disease receives a name and it formally enters the canon of Western Medicine. It then gets circulated in the consciousness of both physicians and patients alike, and we begin to think almost exclusively in terms of disease names, their symptoms, and our identity with those symptoms and diseases. "My asthma is flaring up today," we say; or "my menstrual cramps incapacitate me for days."

When we identify with the disease—usually after receiving a diagnosis—our focus often becomes mitigation of the symptoms that the disease presents. If we address the symptoms well enough, we think, the disease will go away. This orientation to disease management is very different from a commitment to optimal health. For the most part, physicians are taught to be satisfied by a change in the numbers—an adjustment in the lab results—as the measure of health improvement. If your symptoms go away, great! You must be cured! But intuitively we know this isn't the case. We know that our migraines are not caused by an absence of Fiorinal and menstrual cramps are not caused by a deficiency in Motrin. But in the conventional approach to medicine, the "cure" is defined by whatever makes the symptoms go away.

If you have a deep commitment to healing, it is important to understand how conventional mainstream medicine—and most of us—assume healing works. It isn't that allopathy is right or wrong; it's simply a worldview, a frame of reference from which most contemporary physicians do their work. And it is a worldview that has become ingrained in American culture; it has become de facto "normal." Of course, allopathy has profoundly valuable techniques to offer in the service of improving human life, but as the dominant—and for many, the singular—medical paradigm in the United States, it leaves little room for a candid discussion on the true causes of illness and the processes that support optimal health and healing.

Physicians throughout history have used countless other paradigms and world-views when treating their patients. In the Middle Ages, most physicians believed that the body was ruled by four humors, which were responsible for illness when they fell out of balance. Countless schools of thought and traditions have sought to understand and treat human disease using different frameworks. In Traditional Chinese Medicine (TCM)—which is still practiced today throughout the world in the form of acupuncture and herbal remedies—five elements and an intricate system of energy meridians inform both treatment and diagnosis. Ayurveda, homeopathy, naturopathy, osteopathy, chiropractic—these paradigms for health and healing have deep roots in human cultures and can offer profoundly useful techniques in helping you create a life of joy and longevity. Each paradigm has different strengths and no single paradigm is sufficient for treating every individual's health.

Over the course of the subsequent chapters, we'll be looking at many of the common underlying causes that drive symptoms and affect how disease takes hold in the body. We'll also be looking at some of the methods you can use for restoring optimal health, including, but not limited to, the relief of your chronic symptoms. Learning to trust the body's capacity to heal is a journey of healing in and of itself, and when we undertake this process with commitment and integrity, what we receive is not simply improved physical health, but a renewed sense of connection, peace, and contentment.

Chapter Two

Foundations for Health

Most people know that their car oil needs to be changed on a regular basis to keep their engine running smoothly. The tire pressure needs to be checked to keep the tread from wearing prematurely and, of course, the car needs gas to run. Like a car, the human body has a set of foundational systems that keeps our engine going. Understanding these systems and how they affect our health and wellbeing can empower us to be powerful agents in maintaining optimal biological health for our body.

Some of these foundational systems are familiar to us, while others might be off our screen entirely. Most of us have some idea that nutrition plays an important role in our health, but do we know how? For those of us who have been challenged by allergies, we might be aware that our immune system is not as strong as it might be. We don't have to have an academic or deeply scientific knowledge of each system, but understanding its basic needs and functions is a crucial tool in living a joyful life.

Like with cars, sometimes we attend to one biological need in isolation. You can keep pouring oil into your engine, but if the filter doesn't get changed, you're still going to be in trouble sooner or later. Similarly, simply changing the oil won't help you if your wheels are out of alignment. Having a greater awareness of the fundamental operating systems that run our body allows us to choose with greater intention which areas we give attention to and when. We may be making healthy eating choices, but if our digestive system is overburdened or our body is toxic, we may not get the benefit from eating healthy foods.

Moving away from a "problem-fixing" model where we wait until breakdown occurs before we take effective action is at the core of living a healthy and fulfilling life. Many of us wait until our cars breakdown before getting them checked out, but unlike cars, we can't replace our body. While we can make certain physical repairs in some circumstances, it is much more efficient—not to mention cost-effective—for us to deepen our awareness of our body's needs and attend to them steadily over the course of our daily life. When we learn about the needs of our body, we may be inspired to make small or large changes so that our daily life as well as our later years can be spent in optimal health. We can only make those choices, however, once we have a certain set of information and begin to actively listen to the information our body provides for us.

While everyone's body functions with a similar operating system, each of us also has unique biochemical needs and an individual set of genetic predispositions. When we understand our own strengths and weaknesses more clearly, they can guide our focus. We can begin to ask more intelligent questions like, "How can I avoid being subject to the pattern of heart disease in my family?" or "How can I make sure my joints continue to operate well into my old age?" If we know our genetic predispositions from our family background, we can anticipate what our bodies will need, act accordingly, and so minimize the likelihood that we manifest those patterns of disease we inherit from our family.

Many people believe, however, that their health and disease predispositions are hardwired, that if several members of their family had cancer they are guaranteed to get cancer themselves. Similarly, many people who have no history of chronic illness think they may be virtually immune to cancer or heart disease. The truth is that this is not how our bodies work. A predisposition is simply that; a predisposition, not a guarantee. When we understand the interrelated nature of our body's vital systems, we can have more clarity about important daily choices that are presented to us and have more power to create a future in which we are healthy, well, and full of vitality, rather than constantly managing pain and disease symptoms.

First, it's useful to have a rough assessment of your own health. In American culture, we often assume that we're healthy if we're not sick, but does the absence of disease mean that our system is functioning optimally? It may be useful to keep the following questions in mind as you read and reflect on your own state of health:

- Do you wake in the morning feeling rested? Do you get to sleep easily?
- Is your energy stable throughout the day or does it decline in the late afternoon?
- Do you move your bowels every day?
- Is your skin smooth?
- Is your hair falling out?
- Does your body feel cold or chilled easily?
- Are your nails brittle?
- Are your joints flexible?
- Do you get heartburn or gas on a regular basis?
- Do you have regular headaches?
- Can you exercise for 20-30 minutes without pain or discomfort in breathing?
- Do you have allergies?

- If you're a woman, do you have premenstrual symptoms or changes in your breast tissue during menstruation.

What follows is an overview of the foundational systems that support our body's health and some stories that show the power of using these systems to build optimal health in our lives. Each of these foundational aspects of health inform how we understand the whole person. While they are presented here individually, they overlap and interrelate with one another in very important ways.

NUTRITION

While nutrition can seem like a complicated set of conflicting opinions by experts that annoy and confuse any logical person, this book is intended to simplify what you need to know to have your body work optimally. At its most basic level, nutrition has to do with how the foods we eat affect the way our bodies function, age, and break down. Minerals, vitamins, amino acids, and essential fatty acids are all central in supporting your body's optimal functioning, and we get the bulk of these nutrients from the foods we eat. The cells in your body need these nutrients to regulate your vital systems and to build new cells, which then builds new organ tissue. The process by which you consume these nutrients—as well as their quality and quantity—determines much about how your body is able to maintain its vast and complex functions.

While every body has a baseline of nutritional demands that we need to survive, the spectrum of what different bodies need in order to function optimally is vast. Two ways to think about the unique needs of your body are the process of aging from birth until death and your own biochemically specific needs that include your personal and family medical history and predispositions. Our life choices and behaviors contribute to our strengths and weaknesses, and it is important to have an understanding of how your habits either support or impede your body's ability to maintain health over the course of your lifetime.

As we grow from conception to birth, childhood to old age, our nutritional demands vary wildly. For instance, during pregnancy, calcium is critically important in the first trimester as the fetus begins its development. As organs are formed in the second trimester, protein needs are the greater focus, and, in the final trimester, the brain and nervous system are being developed and require specific amino acids and essential fatty acids. Young men and women going through puberty have higher requirements for Zinc, Vitamin A, essential fatty acids, and clean proteins as their hormone levels soar and affect almost every system in the body. As many people age into their later years, hydrochloric acid (HCl) in the stomach decreases. HCl is essential for calcium absorption, which strengthens bones and prevents osteoporosis. Attending to digestive support in older people is essential to ensure they absorb enough calcium and to prevent bone weakness and deterioration. These are just a few examples of how the biological processes of aging require different nutritional adjustments to keep our bodies running optimally. Knowing how to make these adjustments over the course of your life is a key to aging gracefully.

In addition to the normal biological processes of aging, it is also crucial to have an awareness of your own biochemical individuality, your own particular strengths and weaknesses. A person's biochemical individuality is influenced in part by family history, genetics, and early life patterns. Having a familiarity with these variables can make an enormous difference when it comes to supporting optimal health.

Understanding your own particular biochemical needs can help you make easy adjustments in your lifestyle and food habits as they are needed. As life's circumstances change, so do the needs of our bodies. The fluctuating mental and physical demands at work, in our relationships, and in other areas of our lives require us to adjust our intake of healthy proteins and blood sugar-stabilizing foods to help our bodies accommodate different levels of stress. Part of creating and sustaining health is knowing how to adjust our lifestyle and eating habits when the circumstances and demands of our life change. Long-term distress brought on by physical injury, chronic illness, or emotional traumas like divorce, the death of a loved one, or sudden unemployment is extraordinarily taxing on the body, but we can lessen the brunt of the intensity by making specific adjustments in our eating habits. At times, this can simply mean avoiding sugar, dairy, or processed foods. At other times, this might mean getting adequate sleep, drinking more water, or supplementing your diet with certain herbs, vitamins, and medical protein foods that are designed to help the body function optimally.

The difference between knowing how to direct our nutritional needs when our circumstances change and letting nutrition go by the wayside is often the difference between stress and distress. Stress and distress differ because stress is merely the demand we encounter—it is a fundamental part of life that everyone faces. Distress, on the other hand, is when we do not have the capacity to meet the demand in a healthy way. As most of us know, living with chronic distress has physical, emotional, and mental consequences.

One of the consequences we have come to take for granted is "normal aging," by which we expect that increased years in age correlate with increased likelihood of disease and suffering from disease. Having a grounded understanding of our body's changing nutritional needs equips us with the tools to age gracefully and optimize our chances of dying naturally of old age.

The aging process is exacerbated by having an acidic pH in the body, which contributes to the accelerated breakdown of tissues and the increased presence of chronic inflammation. Acidity in the body also makes it much easier for disease to take hold. Eating excess animal proteins, processed sugar, alcohol, white flour, large amounts of coffee, and enduring high levels of distress

---

ACID vs. ALKALINE

Acid and Alkaline refer to the pH of an environment, and is measured on a scale from 1-14. A pH above 7 is considered alkaline (or basic) and a pH below 7 is considered acidic. Pure water has a pH of close to 7. The pH of human blood runs slightly alkaline, from 7.35-7.45, while other fluids in the body can measure more acidic or more basic depending on their function. High levels of acidity in the body—caused by diet and chronic stress—increase inflammation and susceptibility to disease.

---

push the pH of the body into an acidic state. Inflammatory diseases like arthritis, colitis, cancers, and allergies thrive when the human body is too acidic, so taking an active role in alkalizing our body is one of the most effective measures we can take to prevent disease from taking root.

It may not be an oversimplification to say that everyone should eat more alkaline. The reality is that many diseases have a hard time taking hold and progressing in the body when our pH is more alkaline. With a few exceptions, a diet high in fruits and green vegetables and low in animal protein and processed foods helps maintain a pH in the body that is inhospitable to disease.

The direction of nutrition that encourages the body to heal almost always includes alkalization. Either for a period of a few months, or sometimes longer, the body has to reset itself because it has sustained such an acidic state. Abstaining from animal proteins, processed foods, white flour, vinegar, and white sugar while focusing on fruits, vegetables, and whole non-glutinous grains alkalizes the body. Relaxing more, meditating, and laughing also help prevent distress that keeps the adrenal system from working overtime and contributing to the creation of acid byproducts in our system.

ALKALIZATION

Alkalization is the process of keeping the body's internal environment in the ideal pH range. The average American diet is extremely acidic—high levels of processed and refined sugar, processed grains and flour, animal protein, and dairy. Undertaking a food plan that focuses on fresh fruits and vegetables shifts the pH of the body, reducing inflammation and the likelihood of disease.

Knowing how to support our specific nutritional needs takes some investigation. There is no prescription that works for everyone, but there are a number of baseline practices that set the stage for adaptability and vitality throughout life.

Here are some things to consider that affect both the quality and effectiveness of your nutritional intake. Feel free to choose one or two items to focus on per week, and integrate them into your life in a way that feels easy and sustainable.

- Eat more local, organic whole foods.
- Chew your food well when you eat. This supports good digestion and, therefore, absorption.
- Drink four to six glasses of water per day, pure un-chlorinated.
- Eat mindfully, only when you are settled and relaxed.
- Eat food that is seasonally available.
- Minimize refined sugar, white flour, coffee, red meat, dairy, fried foods, salt, alcohol, and processed foods.
- Follow a food plan concentrating on fresh fruits and vegetables every day.

- Eat one to two servings of whole, unprocessed grains, seeds, and nuts.
- Eat more nutrient dense foods, such as leafy green vegetables.
- Graze: Eat three meals per day and two snacks.
- Eat more foods that are raw and less cooked, i.e., foods that are sprouted contain more natural enzymes.

CASE HISTORY
Alleviating Carol's Pre-Menstrual Symptoms with a Healthy Diet

Carol sat across from me, nervously explaining that she thought she might be suffering from split personalities. As soon as her menstrual cycle began, she said, she was like a different person. Her symptoms were severe and over the years had lengthened from seven days to now at least 10 days or 12 days before her flow began. Her breasts became so tender she couldn't jog or hug anyone for nearly two weeks. She painted a picture of a frantic woman who would cry at the least provocation, was hyper critical and sensitive, and very moody when she was not crying or arguing with someone. Carol had three children and a full time job as a schoolteacher and felt like her pre-menstrual symptoms were ruining her life.

Carol was like so many other women who suffer from painful cycles but were never offered the connection between low blood sugar, liver toxicity, and the progesterone/estrogen cycle of a woman's body. After evaluating Carol's particular nutritional strengths and weaknesses, I recommended that she take specific amounts of Vitamin E, Magnesium, Borage Oil, and Lipotrophic Factors, a supplement that would help her liver break down estrogen more efficiently. I asked her not to eat any foods that might have hormonal residue, like chicken, dairy or red meat, as well as to abstain from coffee, alcohol, and white sugar for three months. Instead, I asked her to dramatically increase her fresh vegetable intake and begin drinking fresh vegetable juice through-out the day, and encouraged her to become aware of eating foods that would help alkalize her body.

Three weeks after our first visit, Carol's pre-menstrual symptoms were still severe and long. In the second month however, they had decreased in severity by 50% and lasted only seven days. I added a medical protein food as well as an herbal preparation to support her liver in the very complicated biochemical conversions for estrogen degradation. In the third month, her breast tenderness and moodiness were 20% of what they were and began only two days before her flow. By the fourth cycle, Carol's symptoms were completely gone.

Giving the organs of elimination a rest while using supplements that encourage hormonal balance and immune strengthening is at the heart of the paradigm of detoxing the body. Rather than suppress symptoms, it is important to uncover their biological origin and then tailor a program that will remove the blocks that hinder the body's optimal functioning. In Carol's case, stabilizing her blood sugar, alkalizing her body, and supporting her liver functions helped to balance her hormone cycle. Fundamentally, this approach was grounded in sound nutrition.

BLOOD SUGAR STABILITY
AND THE ADRENAL SYSTEM

Stabilizing blood sugar is a crucial part of optimizing our organ functions and maintaining good health. When we eat complex carbohydrates, they are broken down by the body into the simplest of building blocks called glucose. One glucose molecule is sugar. Two together is called fructose and multiple molecules together is a complex carbohydrate. This is what the cells in our body use for all our basic life processes that require energy. Ideally, our energy is stable throughout the day because our blood sugar is steady. If we need more energy, we either eat more or we use reserves of blood sugar stored in the liver and muscle fibers called glycogen. Most people, however, have mild to moderate low blood sugar—also called hypoglycemia—which can be a precursor to diabetes. For people with a family history of diabetes, hypoglycemia is a red flag. In order for our blood sugar to be properly regulated, our pancreas needs to produce insulin. Insulin signals the cells in our body to pull glucose from the bloodstream so it can be used for energy. However, when we eat irregularly, miss meals, and eat simple sugars, our blood sugar levels vacillate and our pancreas becomes stressed and can't keep up with the demand of making insulin.

Symptoms of low blood sugar you might notice include unstable energy throughout the day, sugar cravings, alcohol intolerance, headaches, and dizziness. If any of the following apply to you, your blood sugar is more than likely on a roller coaster ride throughout the day:

- Frequent consumption of candy, soda, cookies, etc.
- Habitual dieting, binging, or meal missing
- A family history of diabetes
- Moderate to severe allergies

- More than five alcoholic drinks per week
- Significant distress over an extended period of time
- Managed pain for an extended period of time

Each of these predispositions and lifestyle habits can put pressure on the pancreas, reduce glycogen reserves, and seriously compromise our blood sugar stability. Over the course of time, this begins to have a great impact on our organ and tissue functions, our health, and well-being.

If your blood sugar is erratic and has been for years, it's likely that your pancreas, adrenals, and liver are all over stressed. Chronic low blood sugar depletes the body of chromium and B vitamins, which are necessary for the production of insulin and a well-functioning nervous system. If you are hypoglycemic on a regular basis, either from missing breakfast, relying on coffee for energy or eating simple sugars (candy or soft drinks) on the go, your adrenal system is constantly being asked to compensate for the lack of real energy (glucose or glycogen) by supplying adrenaline for a burst of energy. Adrenaline is produced by the adrenal gland, a small pea-shaped organ that sits above your kidneys and is responsible for producing adrenaline and other corticosteroids. It is meant to kick in when the body needs a jolt of energy, as in a fight or flight scenario, but most people have hyperactive adrenal systems from high-stress lifestyles, caffeine reliance, and low blood sugar. Rather than calling on our adrenal system for survival purposes, therefore, people with low blood sugar come to use it as a backup energy system, like a steady drip of energy that slowly depletes our reservoir without replenishment.

If your blood sugar bottoms out on a regular basis and your adrenal system is being called to compensate, it's likely that you often have adrenal overload and fatigue, since the adrenal system isn't designed for constant use. If you have poor vision at night, light bothers you, and you have irritations to your skin and mucous membranes, it's also likely that high adrenal demand is depleting

ADRENAL OVERLOAD

Many people rely on adrenaline to get them through the day. Ongoing stress, excess sugar and alcohol, chronic allergies and other physical symptoms, and emotional overwhelm tax the adrenal system. If our diet is not supporting stable blood sugar and we are not getting enough rest or exercise, our adrenal system becomes "fatigued" from overproduction, and we rely more and more on stimulants like coffee, while still getting tired easily. This may contribute to the development of stress-related diseases such as fibromyalgia, heart disease, arthritis, colitis, and chronic respiratory symptoms.

you of vitamins A, B, and C, which are all used in the production of adrenal hormones. If your gums bleed easily, your hair is thinning or falling out, your allergies are getting worse, you bruise easily, or get late afternoon fatigue these might be indicators that you aren't getting sufficient nutrients to keep up with basic cell maintenance and the increased demand on your adrenal system.

Because adrenaline is an important hormone, a decade or more of an overactive adrenal gland can impact other hormone levels in the body. This can result in hot flashes, low libido, night sweats, and vaginal dryness in perimenopausal and menopausal women. By the time a woman comes to perimenopause or menopause, the adrenal gland, which should have helped her compensate for the diminished levels of estrogen and progesterone, is actually under-producing adrenal hormones that might have eased her symptoms, making menopause a more difficult experience.

For anyone, adrenal overload might result in chronic fatigue syndrome, chronic infections, and exacerbated allergic symptoms, which in turn stress the adrenal system even more. When you have adrenal overload, your body is less able to cope with stress, which is the adrenal system's primary function. Because the excessive demand on your adrenal system depletes the body of vitamins A, B, and C, your immune system no longer has the optimal resources it needs to keep you protected and you are now more vulnerable to infection, developing allergies, and accelerated signs of aging.

It is important to have a broad time line of how your body's systems are functioning. Most breakdowns occur on the scale of months and years, not overnight. If you miss a meal one day and your adrenals kick in to help you out, it won't impact you that much in the long run if you get back to a healthy lifestyle the next day. It is when our lives become habitually frantic, when we miss meals daily and our diet is replete with processed foods and simple sugars, when we become hooked on caffeine—this is when we develop patterns that stress the body's basic functions. Then, we are no longer looking at creating optimal health; we are simply attempting to mitigate breakdown after breakdown.

Addressing blood sugar stability and adrenal overload means looking at what motivates certain habits—not just dietary habits but emotional ones as well. If you habitually skip breakfast and don't take in any real calories until noon—and after two cups of coffee—what would it take to shift that habit? If you eat on the go and rush through your meals, what would it take to eat more mind-fully? If a soda and a bag of chips frequently comprise portions of a meal and you find your energy crashing by the middle of the afternoon, what would it take to introduce more nourishing foods?

The process of stabilizing your blood sugar is an exercise in deeply understanding the origins of your lifestyle and eating hab-its, and then making appropriate adjustments. Attending to your blood sugar is a necessary part of improving your overall health because the status of your blood sugar is intimately connected to almost every process in your body. When your blood sugar is low and your adrenals are forced to compensate, your entire system is stressed, and over a long period of time this can lead to breakdowns in almost every part of your body—in your digestion, skin, circulation, as well as your mental and emotional resources. Stabilizing blood sugar helps reduce adrenal stress, allowing the body's natural functioning to optimize.

Distress is also a kind of behavior that we consider to be a normal part of our experience after a period of years. Changing what we eat is often not sufficient to change how we feel (though it is a big part of how we feel). Consider what chronically burns you out or drives you to overwhelm. What would it take to change your relationship to these aspects of your life? How could they be less taxing? Beginning to notice the origins and belief systems that drive our lifestyle habits is a critical step to finding the power to change them.

So, how do you stabilize your blood sugar if you suffer from hypoglycemia? Fortunately, it's really quite easy. While at first glance the term "blood sugar" might seem to suggest that we need more sugar in our diet, the fact is that simple, processed, and refined sugars actually destabilize our blood sugar level, because the body metabolizes it too quickly. The importance of starting each day with a nutritionally dense breakfast specific to your needs cannot be overstated. For you, this might be a multi-grain cereal or oatmeal with fresh fruit, whereas someone else might need a high energy protein smoothie given their metabolic needs. Then, eating small meals, comprised of healthy foods, throughout the day is the best way to keep a steady influx of nutritionally dense calories coming into your body. Know your specific nutritional status so you can eat foods with the right amount of vitamins and minerals (A, B, C, chromium etc.) that are important for your pancreas and adrenal gland to function optimally. Minimize amounts of sugar and alcohol that challenge insulin demands and deplete your body of necessary nutrients. Snack on healthy power foods—medical protein foods, celery, carrots, apples, hummus, and small amounts of almonds and sunflower seeds—throughout the day. This is the best prevention for hypoglycemia (and, later, diabetes) and adrenal fatigue.

CASE HISTORY
Eliminating Sam's Headaches by Stabilizing Blood Sugar

Sam was a 34-year-old executive running five companies with a total of 120 employees. He came to see me at the request of his wife. Staring out the window of the office overlooking downtown Boston, it was clear he really did not want to be there, and was appeasing his wife by keeping his appointment. Sam was an athlete and a man who derived his sense of identity from high performance and competition. It was very difficult for him to talk about the severe daily headaches that just about incapacitated him. Every day, in the late afternoon, Sam felt like a tight band was wound around his head. On a scale from 1-10, his pain was anywhere from 6-9, 10 being the worst pain he could imagine.

Evaluating Sam was fairly straightforward. He had no heavy metals, no chronic infection, and no allergies. Sam was the image of a man driven by a singular vision of success and money. As a marathon runner, Sam was clocking nearly 75 miles a week between events. Each morning after running, his routine was to skip breakfast, grab a cup of coffee, get to work early, and begin tackling business problems. Sam was a brilliant businessman, but when it came to nutrition and supporting his body to meet the myriad demands he faced each day, he was in the dark. After evaluating his nutrient levels—vitamins, minerals, essential fatty acids, and protein—the picture of what caused Sam's headaches became clearer.

Sam's high-intensity schedule demanded a much steadier stream of energy than his diet and eating habits were supplying. His B vitamins and chromium levels were low, which compromised his insulin production, and he wasn't getting nearly enough amino acids (protein) intake to keep up with his heavy workload and intense exercise schedule. Sam's dry skin and light sensitivity also indicated that he was Vitamin A deficient. From an organ stand-point, it was clear that Sam's adrenal system was overtaxed and he was suffering from adrenal fatigue.

Sam assumed that his headaches were a result of overstress, but I explained the biological importance of eating nutritionally dense foods at regular intervals. Keeping his blood sugar stable would prevent his adrenal system from burning out and depleting the rest of his body. Sam agreed to give me 90 days, and we started him out on a food regimen that included breakfast every morning and snacking on power foods that were packed with nutrients. We eliminated alcohol, white flour, sugar, and added certain herbs and vitamins to help stabilize his blood sugar and build his adrenal gland's capacity.

In 30 days, his headaches had decreased in severity but were still frequent. In the second month, his headaches were much less painful and only happened every other day. By the third month, Sam's headaches were rare and ranged from 1-3 on the pain scale. Sam also learned important skills about stress management. He began to meditate regularly and practice three-minute positive visualizations twice a day. Most importantly, Sam began to cultivate an awareness of how his physical experience, diet, and stress levels were related, which allowed him to make adjustments throughout the week as his work demands fluctuated.

CASE HISTORY
Using a Holistic Approach to Address Don's Depression

Don was a 32-year-old machinist who came to see me for help with his depression. He had broken his arm two months before coming to see me, and the boredom of being out of work with an injury was challenging. Don was a man with virtually no hobbies and few friends. His whole life was his work.

About a month before Don came to see him, his grandmother passed away. She had raised Don since childhood, and the loss was a crippling blow to Don's sense of family and support. Prior to breaking his arm and navigating the emotional upheaval of losing his grandmother, Don had maintained a healthy lifestyle. He ate mostly well, took a multivitamin, and had steady energy throughout the day.

However, when Don broke his arm and had to take a leave of absence from work, he did not make any adjustments to his lifestyle to accommodate the added stress. Taking extra B and C vitamins would have helped his system deal with the increased demand, and taking calcium hydroxyappetite would have helped his bone knit together faster. Bored without work and over stressed by his situation, his eating habits began to deteriorate, leaving him hypoglycemic, dizzy and tired in the afternoons, with frequent bad headaches. I talked to Don about listening to his body and learning to make fine tuned adjustments to his lifestyle that would lessen the physical impact of his stress and grief.

It was also important for Don to have an outlet where he could authentically express his emotional experience. The tumultuousness of his circumstances was understandably challenging, and Don felt he had no recourse other than to "ride it out." I asked Don what it would look like for him to honor and respect his grief, and we found ways for him to make sure he had permission and space to express his feelings of loss and sadness. After working with Don for two months, he felt revitalized. He was taking calcium hydroxyappetite for his bone healing, DLPA and 5-HTP for his depression and brain functioning, and B vitamins and herbs to support his adrenals in dealing with the stress. More importantly, he felt clearer about his purpose and the values that guided his life. He was in touch with a deep gratitude for his grandmother and felt confident that he now had a set of tools he could use to help him make adjustments when the circumstances in his life changed in the future.

Don is an example of a great guy who had multiple traumatic events occur in close succession but didn't have the resources to help his body cope with the increased physical demands of emotional stress. Learning to attend to his body's changing needs helped him cope with the increased stress; he had enough supplemental resources, could attend to his diet, and had a commitment to expressing his feelings in a way that helped him heal from the profound loss he was experiencing.

THE IMMUNE SYSTEM

If you have adrenal overload—which is to say your adrenal glands work overtime to produce more adrenaline as compensation for low blood sugar—it is likely that you have vitamin A, B and C depletion, since these are key ingredients in the construction of adrenaline. Vitamin A and C depletion also significantly impedes a high functioning immune system. So for people who live a high-stress lifestyle and get sick frequently, there is a fairly clear indication that the combination of low blood sugar, high adrenal output, and vitamin A and C deficiency are compromising the immune system's ability to ward off infectious agents and illness.

The immune system is an interrelated network of organs that protect you from both inner and outer antagonists that interrupt optimal efficiency in the body. It is related to the thymus, the spleen, and other lymphatic structures that make white blood cells, which fight infection in the body. The immune system is also intimately related to the nervous system as well as to the body's capacity to deal with stress via the adrenal system.

Here are some of the other factors that indicate whether or not your immune system is compromised:

- High tissue levels of heavy metals such as mercury, lead, and aluminum
- Adrenal fatigue
- Toxicity
- Undetected infectious agents such as Candida albicans
- Allergies and sensitivities

- Insufficient amounts of certain vitamins and minerals that are key to immune function, such as Zinc, vitamins A, C, and D

Few people seem to be aware of the impact of heavy metals on their health, but for some people it can be quite significant. Heavy metals build up in the body over time and are not cleared by the standard methods of excretion (urine, bowel movements, and sweat). They bind nutrients in the digestive system, which blocks absorption and causes stress in the nervous system. If heavy metals are impeding your nutritional absorption, your body doesn't have the basic building blocks it needs to regenerate. As in the previous discussion on low blood sugar, when your body does not have the resources it needs, the system becomes stressed and things begin to break down; we stay sick longer, our allergies stay severe, and our energy levels continue to be low and unreliable.

The ways that heavy metals get into our bodies are myriad and often unseen. For example, cooking food at high heat in aluminum foil or aluminum cookware brings aluminum into the body. Most deodorants use aluminum oxide as an antiperspirant, which then gets absorbed into the body through the skin. Mercury from tuna, swordfish, and other large fish, as well as from dental material are absorbed into the body. If we live in houses with copper water pipes, copper will leak into the water we drink. These days, due to increased awareness and regulation, few people have high lead or cadmium levels, though these were once quite substantial risks in the population.

Heavy metals alone are rarely sufficient cause for poisoning or hospitalization. What is more common, however, is that your chronic health issues—your allergies, chronic low energy, chronic high stress, asthma, skin problems and so on—are all exacerbated by how heavy metals interfere with nutrient absorption.

CASE HISTORY
Reducing Stacy's Candida and Heavy Metals Through Cleansing

Stacy first came to my office in 1983 complaining of headaches and depression that she had suffered from for years. She was a young medical doctor and extremely passionate about her work. Yet, she frequently got sick and found that, no matter what kind of medicine she took, her symptoms persisted for weeks at a time.

I did a full evaluation, looking at her nutritional levels, digestive enzymes, and organ strengths and weaknesses. She had no history of allergies, but tests came back showing a high presence of mercury. Tests also showed an increased amount of an infectious agent called Candida albicans, a naturally occurring fungus that lives in the digestive tract and is perfectly benign at normal levels. At elevated levels, however, candida can cause a host of problems. At the time Stacy came into my office, two physicians, Orian Truss and William Crook, were pioneering research in the different symptoms associated with increased levels of candida. It was already commonly accepted that persistent vaginal discharge, certain skin rashes, and athletes foot were tied to high levels of candida, but Truss and Crook postulated a multitude of other symptoms including headaches, poor digestion, depression, mood swings, increased susceptibility to infection, and allergies all correlated with above average candida levels.

Stacy's high mercury load, in combination with her elevated candida, seemed likely candidates for the source of her symptoms. Reducing heavy metal levels, however, is a somewhat challenging task that takes time. When treating heavy metals, I frequently use a method called chelation. The word "chelate" comes from the Greek and means "to grab onto" or "to claw," and oral chelation seeks to bind heavy metals so they can be transported out of the body using normal routes of elimination. While Stacy's susceptibility to frequent illness and infection began to abate in the first eight weeks, it took close to six months to reduce her mercury levels to a place where they were no longer interfering with optimal immune functioning. Herbs and nutritional supplements helped reduce the frequency and intensity of her headaches, while Stacy also went through several rounds of detoxification to bring her candida back to ideal levels. After 18 months, Stacy felt renewed. Her headaches were rare, and her depression had almost entirely vanished.

*

The immune system is also affected by allergies and sensitivities. By definition, allergies are immediate responses that take place anywhere from a few seconds to a few hours in mild, moderate, or severe reactions to some external stressor—food, inhalants, preservatives, additives, drugs, etc. A sensitivity is a delayed reaction to a stressor that occurs after four hours or after repeated exposure over time; it is not the same thing as a mild allergy. If you have sensitivities, you may have a biochemical reaction to some stressor, but it will not show up immediately as with an allergy. Sensitivities also do not show up in allergy testing; they only show up in sensitivity testing and many allergists are not trained to detect or treat sensitivities. It is common for people to have an undiagnosed food or drug sensitivity with very chronic symptoms, but because the onset of the sensitivity symptoms does not fit the model of an allergy and they have not been tested, many people remain unaware of what causes their symptoms.

Allergies and sensitivities both have the effect of draining the immune system. Chronic allergies and sensitivities deplete the adrenal system, sap our energy, and use up zinc, Vitamin C, and essential fatty acids, which affect the mucus membranes, and the digestive and nervous systems. The unmetabolized chemical effect of constant reactions creates a toxic burden in the body. So, if you are constantly exposed to an irritant that triggers allergic or sensitivity reactions, your immune system is compromised by constant nutritional depletion due to the continuous toxic stress. This is why people with chronic sensitivities and allergies often have very dry skin, dry eyes, and get sick easily and frequently.

Most standard treatments for allergies like asthma and eczema simply address the symptom, not the antagonist; the inhaler may help us breath, but it doesn't cure the asthma, neither does the cortisone cure the eczema. However, allergies and sensitivities can be healed through a process of:

1. Identifying and minimizing the irritant
2. Interrupting the biochemical reactions that are triggered
3. Strengthening the body to become less affected by the irritant.

One of the key nutrients that supports a healthy immune system is zinc, which isn't common in most foods. It can be found in oysters, ginger, and pumpkin seeds, which aren't central in many people's food plans. Unfortunately, zinc is easily depleted in the body by white processed sugar, so most people have suboptimal zinc levels that make their immune systems susceptible. Pandemic low levels of zinc have contributed to a skyrocketing of allergies and sensitivities. It is very difficult to make up for lost zinc through diet, because it is so uncommon in food, and it may be useful to take a zinc supplement while minimizing processed sugar intake.

Vitamin A, on the other hand, is compromised by air pollution and radiation. Yet it is critical to healthy mucus membranes that form the inside and outside of the skin. Vitamin A is also one of the main factors in making adrenalin. For some people with allergies and sensitivities eating more vitamin A rich foods like dark leafy greens can be helpful. For most people, this won't be sufficient to keep up with the demands of the allergic reactions. Zinc and vitamin A are examples of nutritional biochemical factors related to why people have allergies and why they get worse under stress and as they age. Taking a vitamin A supplement, however, should only be done under the guidance of a nutritionally-trained physician, as too much vitamin A can be toxic.

CASE HISTORY
Eliminating Betty's Asthma with Supplements

Betty was 38-years-old when she first came to see me. She loved her life, loved being a mother, and was a devoted community organizer, but she had endured a lifetime of severe asthma and was dependent on her inhalers. In our health review, she mentioned that she had also experienced chronic constipation, gas, and bloating most of her life. After doing a full evaluation, I asked Betty to consider two primary issues related to her Asthma. First, the inhalers did nothing to neutralize the dust and mold that triggered the reaction; the inhalers only forced a response from the body that made her more comfortable during reactions. Because the allergies were so severe, her body was chronically depleted in important nutrients that she needed for normal functioning. Making nutritional adjustments to her diet and having her take specific supplements would help minimize the binding effect her allergic reactions had on nutrient absorption. Then we could separately work on decreasing the frequency of the triggering.

Triggered allergies cause a cascade of biochemical reactions that deplete the body of vital nutrients. Reactions use up vitamin C and vitamin A to deal with the stress of the reaction. Your body then no longer has the sufficient resources it expects to have for its other vital processes. Betty agreed to a nutritional program of foods and supplements that included large amounts of buffered vitamin C, beta carotene, zinc and vitamin B6. Second, I wanted Betty to appreciate that her immune system and lung capacity were compromised by some food sensitivity and a lifetime of poor digestion. Food sensitivities can impact hydrochloric acid levels in the stomach, which can mean that proteins are not broken down completely, resulting in a pattern of sluggish bowel movements and chronic bloating.

It was important to get Betty's digestive process and bowel movements regular to see if that had any impact on her lung capacity and breathing challenges. After a few months of taking an HCl supplement before eating, Betty's bowels became daily and her bloating and gas were completely eliminated. When I told her that in Traditional Chinese Medicine, the lungs and the large intestine where energetically related, she was not surprised that her asthma symptoms and allergic reactions had improved by 75% simply through addressing her digestion.

CASE HISTORY
Addressing Bobby's Eczema, ADD, and Allergies with a Healthy Diet

Bobby was eight when his parents brought him in to see me. As a baby, he had terrible colic and developed eczema at three months old, but topical cream treatment had no effect. As Bobby got older, his parents noticed that he was socially uncomfortable around other kids and seemed to twitch a lot. He had been diagnosed with ADD, but the side effects of his medication were severe and his parents did not notice an improvement in his focus, listening skills, or attention. Bobby also had many allergies and food sensitivities, some of which his parent's knew about, others that remained to be diagnosed.

Working with Bobby revealed that his nervous system did not like any preservatives, chemicals, pesticides, or additives. Moreover, Bobby was very low in zinc, gamma linolenic acid, omega 3s and vitamin A—the toll on his immune system from his allergies was large.

I made sure that Bobby felt he could trust me and asked him to be truthful with me and his mom about how challenging it was for him not to eat the foods that triggered his allergies. He tearfully responded how hard it was for him to be so different from other kids his age. We began to play a game where he would count the different colors the he ate during the day and then tell me about them. I asked him not to eat anything colored white, promising to reintroduce his favorite foods when it was safe to do so. As we began to build our trust together, Bobby was more willing to eat foods he didn't like, understanding that his taste buds might grow to like them and that they would help his skin to stop itching. Slowly, he began to enjoy eating veggies with flax seed oil and brown rice. We used organic fruit smoothies to satisfy his sugar cravings, and medical foods designed with high-grade proteins helped repair his tissues and keep his blood sugar even. He took homeopathic antigens and a handful of supplements every day for six months that his mother crushed into powder and mixed into apple sauce.

Bobby's willingness to try new things, make deals about food, and be supported to feel better was incredible and inspiring. After six months, he was transformed, relaxed, and calm. His skin was smooth and he had no itchy symptoms. His parents were happy that he was listening to them more, while his teachers and friends enjoyed his company at school. After six months, we began reintroducing some of the foods Bobby had refrained from eating. He was able to eat soy, eggs, small amounts of refined sugar, and some dairy, though never more than two of these foods on the same day. Gluten and wheat products were introduced more gradually after eight months. We kept the bulk of Bobby's diet focused on healthy fresh vegetables and non-glutinous grains with some fish and chicken.

When Bobby first came into my office, he and his parents were clear that he had ADD, as his doctors told him. After learning about how his body responded to different foods, neither Bobby nor his parents now think of him as having behavioral issues. He is mindful of what he eats and how often, and he has strong relationships with his family and his peers. Removing the antagonists from his diet for a period of time allowed Bobby's immune system to reset itself and stop expending so much of his body's nutrients warding off perceived threats. Then, we were able to retrain his body's response process, which, in conjunction with new habits, allowed him to live a healthy and happy life without the austerity of a permanently strict diet.

CASE HISTORY
Improving Tom's Lung Function with Detoxing

Tom was in his 70s, retired, and suffered for years from chronic lung problems. While he had struggled with weight in midlife, his primary concern was his difficulty breathing. When we first met, I asked Tom to consider that his lung symptoms were related to his allergies and some chronic infections that kept returning despite long-term continual use of antibiotics. His body was toxic with chemicals and pesticides that were being held in his tissues and were depleting his immune system. We put together a detailed program including specific amounts of Vitamin C, B6, N-acetyl cysteine (an amino acid), and herbs like Pleurisy Root and garlic.

We alternated three weeks of guided cleansing and detoxing protocols for his lungs with a month of eating fresh healthy food without dairy, red meat, alcohol, or white sugar. Tom looked 10 years younger after his first three months, and his breathing was improved to the extent that he could go off his inhalers and other synthetic medications. Tom's case is an example of how embedded infections and latent toxicity that is not eliminated from the body can suppress the immune system in specific ways. Clearing these toxins and providing his organs of elimination with extra support helped remove the allergic antagonists from Tom's body so he could breathe better.

THE DIGESTIVE SYSTEM

The digestive system can be broken down into three processes: ingestion, digestion, and absorption. Ingestion relates to the content of what we eat and how we eat it; are we taking in nutrient rich foods like fresh vegetables and fruits? Or are we taking in nutrient-poor food, processed preservatives and lots of refined sugar? Do we eat on the go, erratically, or when we are upset? Is our food grown organically or does it have chemical residue? Additionally, the kind of food we need changes over time. Are we using food therapeutically to rejuvenate specific organ function? Or are we in basically good health and simply using food to maintain homeostasis? These are important questions to look at when simply examining the food we ingest and take into our bodies.

The primary challenge of ingestion lies in the density of nutrients in what you eat. Most people eat for taste, not for the nutritional content. Taste, however, is a conditioned tendency that we develop over the course of our lifetime; it is influenced by our upbringing, environment, culture, and experience. Sometimes we eat based on emotional associations, what feels and tastes like home, or what reminds us of a certain time. Few of us eat in order to support our liver function or to strengthen our adrenals, and even when we do "eat healthy," many of our choices are based on myth and misunderstanding, as if everyone should be a vegetarian (for health reasons) or no one should ever eat sugar. When we think about healthy choices for ingestion, we often think in terms of extremes, and people can get very dogmatic about what's good or bad for their body.

When you use food to create optimal health, there may be foods that you stay away from for a period of time. What to eat in order to get your organs working optimally when they are stressed or diseased is very different from what to eat in order to keep them working brilliantly once they're in top shape. How we eat is as important as what we eat, and developing habits that allow us to ingest food in a mindful and centered way can have a profound impact on our overall health and wellbeing.

What most people eat is nowhere near as nutritionally dense for what they need in order to age gracefully, reduce inflammation, or attend to whatever health goal they might have. So, what goes in our mouths is often less than ideal. On top of that, the second part of the process—digestion—is often compromised by how we eat. Do you eat quickly? Do you multitask while you eat or eat standing up or in your car? Do you eat while you're upset?

The digestive enzymes we use to break down our food in the stomach and the enzymes excreted by the pancreas are all governed by the parasympathetic nervous system. The parasympathetic nervous system and sympathetic nervous system are both a part of the autonomic nervous system, which governs things like digestion and stress, but only one can be active at a given time; the two are competitive. The sympathetic nervous system (of which the adrenals are a part) is turned on (even slightly) when we eat standing up, quickly, while we're in the car, anytime we're multitasking, or emotionally distressed. So, if the sympathetic nervous system is active, the parasympathetic nervous system doesn't send the message to release the digestive enzymes, as it assumes you are otherwise occupied. This can result in gassiness (flatulence), undigested food, nutritional malabsorption, and, consequently, low energy, because your enzymes are not available to break your food down properly.

In addition, not chewing your food means the surface area of your food is greater, because more remains unchewed, and therefore requires more enzymes to break down, which can also reduce absorption. Drinking while you eat can dilute the enzymes in the stomach, making digestion and absorption more difficult. Digestion begins in the mouth—we actually have digestive enzymes in our saliva that begin to break down the food we eat. When we don't chew sufficiently, the enzymes in our mouth don't have a chance to begin the digestive process.

Digestion addresses the breakdown of food matter in our stomach and small intestine. The parietal cells that line the stomach wall secrete hydrochloric acid (HCl), which, in conjunction with enzymes from the pancreas, help to break down food into its most basic constituent elements: from macro-nutrients like protein, fat, and carbohydrates, to micro-nutrients like vitamins, minerals, amino acids, and essential fatty acids. When we talk about digestion, we are asking how competently the HCl and pancreatic enzymes are breaking down food. Because of a lifetime of demand from eating excess animal protein, elderly people can often have diminished levels of HCl in their stomachs, which means food is not completely digested properly. These patients often suffer from gas, bloating, and distension, as well as an inability to absorb minerals like calcium, which is HCl dependent.

As soon as digested food leaves the stomach, passes through the small intestine, and reaches the large intestine, healthy bacterial flora that live in the large intestine ensure that the nutrients from our food are absorbed properly. However, for many people, this process can be very compromised, and the crucial step in ensuring that nutrients are absorbed into the body is significantly undermined. For instance, people who eat very little fiber or drink very little water and are dehydrated over years can erode nutrient absorption by decreasing transit time from ingestion to elimination. People who overuse antibiotics can also significantly reduce healthy bacteria, which allows candida overgrowth. Even if you eat nutrient rich food, you might get very little benefit from it if the flora aren't present in your intestine or are blocked from doing their job of transporting the nutrients through the intestinal lining into your bloodstream. Competitive microorganisms like viruses, parasites, and candida can interfere with ideal absorption of nutrients by diminishing or inhibiting flora in your large intestine. Healthy beneficial flora can be encouraged by eating foods that are fermented or cultured like sauerkraut, yogurt, kefir, miso, or by taking a high quality supplement.

The entire digestive process needs to be evaluated in order to understand how food intake supports optimal or suboptimal organ functioning in the body. Most people, for instance, have never been tested for transit time—the time food takes from ingestion to elimination—and many people who move their bowels daily eliminate food they ate three days ago, which is another form of constipation, rather than eliminating what they ate in the previous eight to 18 hours. Regular and consistent elimination, however, is one of the fundamentals of good health because if the bowel is stagnant, toxins build up and create acidity in the body. Our diet-obsessed culture has convinced many of us that simply restricting or enhancing broad categories of food—carbohydrates, fats, or proteins—will positively impact our bodies, but this mindset neglects the nuances both of individual foods and the specific components of the digestive process.

So, how do you evaluate whether or not your digestive system is functioning optimally? One way to evaluate your digestive functioning is by looking at your symptoms. If you have:

- Heartburn
- Bloating
- Excessive gas
- Constipation
- Chronic loose stools
- Pain in your abdomen
- Bad breath
- Or if certain foods give you headaches and other symptoms that you find uncomfortable

These are all symptoms of a breakdown somewhere in your digestive system. Compromised digestion, however, is not always obvious. Someone could have very poor absorption and the manifestation might be arthritis, chronic infections, or a multitude of other symptoms.

Functional digestion begins with healthy eating habits, which have as much to do with how you eat as what you eat. For optimal health, consider adopting some of the following practices when you eat and your body will have an easier time processing and using the food you eat.

- Take a moment to reflect and center yourself before you eat. This allows the parasympathetic nervous system to turn off, the sympathetic nervous system to turn on, and trigger the release of digestive enzymes.
- Do not eat in moving vehicles or while you're rushing, stressed, or upset.
- Chew your food slowly and thoroughly when you eat.
- Only drink fluids 30 minutes before or after eating, not with food, unless you're taking supplements with your food.
- Take pleasure in the process of preparing food for yourself.

CASE HISTORY
Addressing Mary's Psoriasis through Detoxing

Mary came to see me when she was a junior in college. She had significant skin lesions that her MD told her was psoriasis. After a full nutritional evaluation, I talked to Mary about her lifelong habit of infrequent bowel movements, her high levels of mercury from eating too much tuna, and her chronic dehydration from rarely drinking water. She agreed to do a 21-day cleanse, which we supplemented with replenishing probiotics (flora), essential fatty acids, zinc, and homeopathics, which rejuvenated her digestive capacity for absorption. I had Mary spend another month eating very minimal animal protein, no dairy, alcohol, or sugar, and after three months her psoriasis was 80% improved. Three months after that, it had healed completely. Mary is a perfect example of how interrelated the organs of elimination are with other essential body processes. Over the course of years, Mary's bowels had become toxic and were no longer moving impurities out of her body efficiently. Detoxing her colon in conjunction with a few lifestyle changes allowed her organs of elimination to restore themselves, thereby allowing the rest of her body to function more optimally.

THE STRUCTURAL SYSTEM

Spinal health is one of the most important—and one of the most frequently overlooked—aspects of our overall health. The spine is what allows signals from our brain to reach the rest of our body, so when the spine is compromised, our organs and muscles are also compromised. Most people know that the spine runs the length of the body—from the brain stem into the cervical spine in the neck to the thoracic spine in the mid back, the lumbar spine in the lower back, and down to the sacrum beneath the waist into the tail bone. More than simply adding stability to our skeletal structure, it houses an elaborate network of nerves that carry messages at lightning speed from our brain to the rest of our body.

Every day, our musculoskeletal system can be distressed by poor posture, repetitive body motion leading to excessive wear and tear, sports injuries, chronic inflammation from organ dysfunction, and unresolved emotional and mental experiences that can put pressure on the muscles around the spine and manifest in severe chronic back and neck pain. Over time, the muscles in the neck and back contract, but never release, which builds pressure on the spine and can cause subtle shifts in the vertebrae called subluxations. Subluxations can put pressure on the nerves that the spine is responsible for protecting. For example, in some people this might manifest in sciatica—antagonism against the sciatic nerve that runs from the bottom of the spine into our legs—while others may experience tingling and numbness in their extremities from other blocked nerve signals. For still others, the effects of spinal misalignment and compromise manifests not in pain but in a weakened immune system, poor digestion, allergies, and so on.

Spinal health is not simply about preventing back pain. Each of the vertebrae is associated with nerves traveling into our organs. The nerve at L4 in our lower back, for instance, feeds the uterus in women, which, if the muscles are really contracted, can greatly affect dysmenorrhea (menstrual cramps). Like nutrient absorption, spinal health is one of the barriers to entry, so to speak, before more targeted treatments can be truly effective in creating optimal health in your life. Like many of the models discussed in this section, the best way to approach spinal health is through prevention: many exercise activities like yoga, Pilates, specifically designed stretching programs help build core muscles and keep the spine protected and youthful, while regular spinal adjustments by a trained physician can ensure proper spinal alignment, which in turns supports optimal nerve functioning along the vertebral column.

Because the spine is responsible for sending signals throughout the entirety of the body, the health and integrity of the spine are directly related to aging well. The Erector Spinae muscle on either side of the spine can get very tight, especially under stress. It is important to stretch regularly to keep this muscle flexible, supple, and non constricting on your spine. Putting your body in certain Hatha yoga postures can have profound positive effects on the health and function of the spine and, therefore, the entire function of your body. Some Yoga teachers are extremely talented in using specific yoga postures to rejuvenate and support certain organs to function much more effectively, while strengthening core muscles to support spinal alignment and keep the vertebrae safe.

When you appreciate the central role your spine plays in how your body functions, you will know how important it is to focus on the health of your spine, maintain a strong core (abdominal muscles) and maintain good posture. Ideal posture may be reflected in how you sit in a chair, how you stand up, how you walk or run, and how relaxed your head sits on top of your shoulders. It is very common to carry tension in our neck and shoulder area, and months and years of not releasing this tension can pull our whole body forward which interrupts the nerve signals in the spine and can accelerate aging. Furthermore, because of how we eat, our vertebras can become arthritic, and the openings where our nerves travel to our organs can become narrow, which can diminish nerve impulses from flowing effectively. Following a food plan that's less acidic and knowing how to neutralize distress in your life can help you avoid becoming arthritic as you age and thereby ensure that your organs receive the information they need from your nerves.

CASE HISTORY
Addressing Alice's Chronic Back Pain with Chiropractic Therapy and Nutritional Supplements

Alice came into my office for her follow up appointment. She had had a double mastectomy years earlier and was seeing me as a patient to address ongoing chronic back pain, leg pain, and general low energy. While I took down her medical history during our first visit, I began to think she might have significant structural issues that were impacting her spine, so I asked her to see a chiropractor colleague of mine who I knew to be an extremely talented healer and physician. He found several of the vertebral discs in her low back had significant degeneration, which can occur when the spine is out of alignment for long periods of time. It was clearly the result of a long-standing issue, but this was the first she had heard of her disc degeneration. Despite seeing many medical doctors for years, all she had ever received for her back pain was medication.

When she returned to see me for her next visit, she was exasperated. Why hadn't her other physicians told her more about her structural health or suggested she see a chiropractor? She had been dealing with the same set of symptoms for years but only now felt that she was receiving information that correlated to her experience. After six spinal alignment adjustments, the pressure on her vertebral discs was relieved, creating the opportunity for healing. In a very short period of time, her chronic low back and leg pain was diminished, and her energy began to return. With the support of some nutritional supplements to rebuild her disc and occasional follow-up spinal adjustments, Alice was able to completely regain her energy and sense of stability. She was no longer irritable from managing constant pain and felt like a huge weight had been lifted from off her shoulders.

TOXICITY

As toxins build up in the body and cause higher acidity and organ stress, the body responds with higher levels of inflammation, nutrient malabsorption, reduced energy, and accelerated aging. Detoxing seeks to remove hindrances to the body's natural optimal functioning and alleviates the chronic inflammation, constipation, and allergies that we have come to expect as normal. Chronic inflammation due to toxic build-up is one of the primary causes of compromised organ function, and eating alkalizing foods helps balance the extremely acidic condition that produces inflammation. In any detox protocol—regardless of what foods, juices, or herbs are used—the primary goal is to improve how the organs of elimination—the liver, skin, kidney, lung, and colon—function. We do not have to wait for disease to present itself through dire symptoms before we take measures to improve how our body eliminates toxins.

Detoxing is important because our bodies can be burdened, stressed, and toxic from a number of environmental and lifestyle factors. Pollutants and contaminants in the air, heavy metals, food additives and preservatives, pesticides, metabolic waste, drug residue, alcohol and tobacco, synthetic hormones, and allergens all find their way inside our system, but don't necessarily find their way out quite as easily. Have you ever thought that your body has to deal with a lot more chemicals than when your grandparents were young? It's only since the 1950s that thousands of preservatives, chemicals, and additives have been added to our food and environment. In the last several decades, antibiotics have also been added to our food, while the quantity of both recreational and prescribed drugs is vastly more ubiquitous than only two generations ago.

And this trend is only increasing. It's also no surprise to us that the quality of the air and water is more contaminated from industrial pollutants and petroleum burning. The demands on our body to deal with, metabolize, and eliminate contaminants, chemicals, and toxins is far greater than it was as little as ten years ago and exponentially greater than it was two generations ago.

*

Our bodies are incredible machines, built specifically with routes of elimination as a necessary part of overall health. Our organs have highly specialized functions that—when in optimal condition— work in perfect unison to retain what we need from our food and environment while eliminating what we don't need. Here are the primary ways your body eliminates toxins:

- The liver processes toxins and metabolic waste for removal.
- The lungs filter the air we breathe, allowing the elements we need to reach our bloodstream.
- The kidneys filter fluids and ensure that our cells are hydrated, while keeping our blood clean.
- The colon processes solid waste and absorbs the nutrients we need from our food.
- The skin expels toxins through sweat and keeps our bodies protected from the elements.

When our bodies are unencumbered by toxic burden and stress, they perform magnificently and allow us to experience life with greater ease.

It is important to remember that the body is built to deal with a certain level of toxicity and waste as a natural part of its functioning. But when we become so chronically toxic and overburdened, and especially over long periods of time, vital functions become compromised and we begin to see the symptoms of disease.

The detox model is a foundation for optimizing organ function and health because it is based on the rationale that more toxins go into the body than come out, and over time this develops precursors for disease. For instance, many people assume it is normal to move their bowels every other day; many doctors believe this is normal as well. "Normal" in this instance more accurately reflects the prevalent condition in most patients rather than the "ideal" condition. The same issues can be said of sweat. It is important to both replenish and eliminate fluids from the body on a regular basis. Dehydration and lack of aerobic exercise also compromise the kidneys ability to filter fluids and diminish the lungs' capacity. Although many assume sweat is only a byproduct of exercise rather than a necessary bodily function to eliminate toxins, many people go months or years without sweating.

When we begin to understand precisely how our habits, lifestyle, and accumulated toxic burden from the environment impact specific functions in our body, practices like exercise, healthy eating, and periodic cleansing are no longer social or moral mandates that contribute to our guilt if we don't adhere to them; they become a natural part of how we understand why our bodies function the way they do. Taking care of ourselves then becomes a natural expression of being connected to our bodies.

CASE HISTORY
Avoiding John's Hip Replacement with a Healthy Diet

John was a 40-year-old executive who walked into my office using a cane to support himself. His doctors had told him he needed a double hip replacement, news that was devastating because his passion in life was golf. John lived to play golf and was desperate to avoid the surgery, which would all but cripple his game. Coming to me was a last resort, and as he stared out the window of my office, he casually stated that he did not believe I could help him.

I immediately knew I could help John for two reasons. First, he was about 55 pounds overweight, and I impressed upon him how much that extra weight burdened the joints in his body. Second, John's diet was extremely acidic and damaging to the tissues in his body. He drank coffee on an empty stomach in the morning, ate virtually no vegetables, and relied almost exclusively on animal proteins like roast beef, hamburger, and tuna fish for his meals. The acidic environment that an all-animal protein diet creates in the body can cause extreme inflammation and even arthritis. Treating the arthritis in John was straightforward in my estimation. I asked John to commit to learning about how he could transform his health in 90 days. So great was his desire to avoid surgery that he agreed and committed to following my guidance 100%, no matter how unreasonable it might seem.

John traveled the country three to four days a week for business and decided to buy a small second suitcase so he could bring a juicer and blender with him wherever he went. I had him drink a pint of fresh mixed vegetable juice every day as well as an alfalfa supplement and protein supplement to help alkalize his body. When possible, I found him an organic health food restaurant in the cities he visited for business. In the first month, John lost 18 pounds, 12 pounds in the second month, and 14 pounds in the third month. John said he felt better than he had in 20 years and had no pain when he walked. He maintained his weight loss, never had a hip replacement, and after four months of seeing me had returned to his passion and was playing a round of golf three to four days a week.

Fundamental to John's success was developing a positive attitude. At the beginning of our work, I gave him a copy of Norman Cousin's book *Anatomy of an Illness,* in which he narrates his experience of having an "incurable" condition called ankylosing spondylitis, a collagen wasting disease that can severely diminish mobility. In his determination to overcome his disease, Cousins watched Laurel and Hardy shows to keep his spirits high, as he would laugh through the entirety of the episode. John resonated with the experience of having negative expectations put upon him by his doctors, but was always honest and earnest in his commitment to create a breakthrough in possibility for himself. Reading Cousin's book was a mirror for him that allowed him to take a more active role in his healing experience while we looked at specific strategies to improve his health. By the time we finished working together, not only was John's body transformed, so was his experience of life.

Chapter Three

Nothing ever goes away until it teaches us
what we need to know.

— PEMA CHODRON

To love oneself is the beginning of a lifelong
romance.

— OSCAR WILDE

Love Your Body

I graduated from naturopathic school in 1978 and then practiced for several months in Boulder and San Francisco before returning to the National College of Naturopathic Medicine in Portland as the Director of Development. Though I was happy to be serving the naturopathic community in Oregon, I had always dreamed of returning to Boston to work with Dr. Billotte, since he was my inspiration for pursuing medicine. Finally, in the spring of 1980, I moved back to Boston to begin my practice.

By the summer, two important things had happened that marked a turning point in my life. First, Dr. Billotte, who was already in his 80s, passed away and I never had the chance to work with him as I had dreamed. Second, I had a waiting list six months long for new clients seeking an initial consultation. It was clear to me that the desire for an integrated approach to healing was in high demand, so I asked a dear friend of mine from naturopathic school to come work with me and, together with three other colleagues, we formed the New England Family Health Center.

The health center became a hub for holistic healing in the Boston area. We offered individual medical consultation as well as a spectrum of workshops and classes taught by some of the best thinkers and authors from around the world. Pioneers in the field of nutrition like Jeff Bland and author Dan Millman spoke on integrating spirituality, while teachers like Virginia Fidel introduced hundreds to the role of meditation and healing. It was an exciting time and the health center was a magnet for revolutionary thinking in the realm of health and well-being.

I had come to see that the scientific and anatomical functions of the body alone did not account for good health. Human beings have a vast array of emotional, psychological, and spiritual needs that intersect with one another in meaningful ways and need to be considered alongside the physical indicators of health. So I designed the LOVE YOUR BODY program, a 21-day detox healing workshop, which became a structured ongoing opportunity for clients to inquire into the nature of health and healing in their own lives. In the last 32 plus years, more than 10,000 patients have been through the program, and it has changed as I have continued to grow, learn, and deepen my own health and healing practices.

Although there are books written in the 18th and 19th century describing detox protocols using different foods and herbs, "detoxing" and "cleansing" programs have dramatically increased in popularity over the last decade. The work that I did with Dr. Billotte laid the foundation for me to create a workshop where people could be on a team and accomplish results beyond anything they could do on their own. While a number of recently popular books and pamphlets accessible in health food stores and on the Internet point to a growing legitimacy of detoxification, it remains a therapeutic modality that requires proper guidance.

The LOVE YOUR BODY program is not a one-size-fits-all experience. It is important that each person be evaluated individually and have their detoxification regimen tailored to their specific biochemistry. For those who crave sugar and get sleepy in the afternoon, for instance, accommodating blood sugar is of great importance. The basics of the program, however, are the same. Using seasonally available organic vegetables with small amounts of fruits, and occasionally small amounts of non-gluten grains, we combine medical protein foods that are designed to alkalize the body and detox certain organs, restoring them to their optimal functioning.

Resting the digestive system and encouraging the organs of elimination to work more efficiently can result in very specific improved health and well-being outcomes. Despite the benefits, however, there are several very important caveats to cleansing properly. For instance, not easing into a cleanse by transitioning into it gradually, rather than going immediately from a normal diet of dairy, meat, coffee, and sugar can make the first few days or week of a cleanse enormously difficult. Then, when the cleanse is complete, coming off of a cleanse too quickly and not re-introducing certain foods slowly can undermine all positive results you experience from the cleanse. In addition, if your lifestyle includes prescribed medication, recreational medications, alcohol, or if your body has signs of toxicity, you might want to focus very specifically on certain organs with certain foods and herbs when you cleanse and do a detox. Many popular generic cleanses do not take into account your specific needs and therefore you won't receive the targeted attention your body requires.

There is also the possibility that as the cleanse progresses, you will successfully be eliminating toxins, which will in fact exacerbate your symptoms or develop new symptoms. Remember, your body eliminates toxicity not just through your digestive system, but through your skin, lungs, liver and kidneys. During the course of the cleanse then, while your body is detoxing, your tongue may get coated, you may get headaches, your skin may break out, your bowel functions might change, you might get gassy or bloated, you may find more mucus in the back of your throat, and so on. All of these are common elements to a detoxification process that you must know how to navigate before you assess that the cleanse is not working. It may in fact be working quite well and your body is simply responding to the toxin elimination process.

Core to the LOVE YOUR BODY experience is offering people the opportunity to observe and listen to their body with a new set of distinctions. Different processes, visualizations, and group exercises allow participants to move from judgment and criticism of their body into compassion and connection. The workshop is designed to have you experience yourself as a trustworthy and confident healer, capable of producing levels of well being beyond your rational expectations.

In the context of doing a cleanse for healing—not just to physically detox our organs—many of the emotional or psychological issues that we have with food might arise, sometimes in very challenging ways. The opportunity of a holistic cleanse then, is not simply to heal the body, but to heal those emotional and energetic parts within us that do not serve our well being. A rigorous cleansing process offers us the opportunity to really become aware of our relationship with food and eating, which is a process that few of us ever undertake over the course of our lives. The real benefit of an integrated cleansing process comes not only from temporarily resting and restoring our body by targeting our diet for a short period of time, but from transforming our relationship to food and eating, such that the rest of our lives are spent living with conscious awareness about the interconnected nature of food, our bodies, and our internal experience.

Most people spend so much of their lives tolerating suboptimal health that the results of a 21-day intensive guided cleanse like the LOVE YOUR BODY program are transformative. Their headaches disappear, their distress almost completely vanishes, they have more energy than they can ever remember, greater stamina, smoother skin, a decrease in allergies, a balanced menstrual cycle, and a reduction in all kinds of inflammatory states. And yet the true transformation each individual experiences is a deeply personal one. Participants complete the program feeling profoundly more connected to their confidence and more empowered to live a life guided by healing, having released the negative emotional and mental patterns that are no longer serving them. The intention of the LOVE YOUR BODY program is in the name—that we discover and recover a deep love for our body and for our lives.

CASE HISTORY
Eliminating Jane's Chronic Urinary Tract Irritations Through Detoxing

Jane was a 42-year-old lawyer who came to see me for her relentless urinary tract irritations that had plagued her for seven years. Her doctor diagnosed her with interstitial cystitis and told her that there was no cure and that, other than being on constant antibiotics, he knew of no treatment. The diagnosis left Jane feeling powerless, and the constant antibiotics gave her vaginitis and a terrible upset stomach. While the burning symptoms abated on occasion when she was on antibiotics, the constant discomfort of the side effects made antibiotic treatment unsustainable.

After a complete nutritional evaluation, I found that Jane had high levels of aluminum and mercury in her body, a number of vitamin and mineral imbalances, and an increased level of candida. Steroids, birth control, sugar, excess alcohol, and continual antibiotic usage can cause normal amounts of candida to proliferate into abnormal levels and cause interference in many different organ systems. Her doctor never mentioned that she might take a probiotic supplement to replenish the healthy flora that the antibiotics were destroying in her intestinal tract. The long-term usage of antibiotics had impaired Jane's ability to absorb nutrients through the digestive process and left her depleted.

As I worked with Jane, I kept evaluating different aspects of her symptoms, using food, homeopathics, probiotics, and different nutritional supplements. There were many different variables that needed attention in order to rebuild her immune system, digestive system, and detox the toxic elements from her candida and heavy metals. In six months, Jane did four 21-day LOVE YOUR BODY cleanses, and we replaced the chemical antibiotics with herbal antibiotics when she felt her symptoms were becoming acute. In the first three months, her urinary tract symptoms became milder but still bothered her half the week. In the second three months, she was mostly symptom free but would have twinges of burning a few days per month.

When we completed our work together, Jane was exuberant. She had been symptom free for months, but more importantly she felt confident that she now had a set of tools that could support her ongoing healing. It has been 25 years, and I still see Jane for follow up from time to time, but she has had no recurring urinary tract symptoms. She is a great example of wanting more for herself than being told that her symptoms were just not curable. She never gave up on herself and created breakthroughs in how she experienced life by learning more about the interconnected nature of her body's systems.

In my experience, clients have the most success when they are empowered to be co-collaborators in creating great health for themselves. This requires a strong measure of commitment. Making powerful, specific goals and grounding them in a deep love and appreciation for your body is a vital step toward healing, but, surprisingly, many people never ask what they really want from their health. Are you absolutely certain about what you want? Are you

Health and Healing Exercise

Sit comfortably and in an upright position, preferably in a quiet area. Allow your attention to rest naturally on the breath and notice when it slows or deepens of its own accord. Let yourself simply be present for a moment with the breath with no need to change or alter anything. Simply enjoy resting. Notice if a calm arises spontaneously and allow that relaxation to permeate through the body, or simply stay with the easy rhythm of breathing.

After a few minutes, or whenever you feel ready, pick up a pen and write "My Body" at the top of a clean page. On the next line, write "My Goals."

Write down very specific measurable goals regarding your body and how you relate to it. Perhaps you would like to learn more about what your body needs to continue working well; perhaps you'd like to recover some aspect of your body that doesn't function the way you would like it to; or perhaps you'd just like to sleep more soundly at night. Goals don't have to correct perceived "mistakes," they simply need to be specific. If you can't think of anything in specific, perhaps getting clear about your goals in the coming days is the goal you write down.

Next, write down some action items that will help you reach these goals. Look back over what you've written, and at the bottom of the page write "I LOVE MY BODY!"

committed to achieving it? The Universe responds to clear, intentional, specific requests. If you are ambiguous in your intention, you will receive ambiguity in your outcome. Be clear about your intention, commit to your goals, and move from a place of love for your body.

Chapter Four

To realize that our knowledge is ignorance,
This is a noble insight.
To regard our ignorance as knowledge,
This is mental sickness.
Only when we are sick of the sickness
Shall we cease to be sick.
The Sage is not sick, being sick of sickness;
This is the secret of health.

—LAO TZU (JOHN C.H. WU TRANS.)

Foundations of Healing

Healing is distinct from health. Health, we might say, is a moment-to-moment barometer of our life-sustaining systems. It reflects both how we are feeling...and how our organs are functioning. Healing, on the other hand, is more of a dynamic process through which we identify, express, and release the blocked energy that inhibits our sense of connection to ourselves, others, and the world around us. This is in fact a natural part of life. Trusting our capacity to heal begins first by recognizing healing as an inborn part of who we are, not simply what we do. Every one of us is a healer. Stepping more fully into this state of being is one of the most powerful intentions we can have.

> # SPACE
>
> Space is related to peace, presence, and non-attachment. It refers to a state of being beyond rationality where healing and creativity take place. It arises when we are connected to the depth of our being, free from the busy preoccupations of the mind.

While healing does promote our physical health, it also opens up possibilities for us to be in communication with different aspects of ourselves and brings us a greater level of connection with life. This healing connection can be enormously powerful for developing inner peace and creativity, finding resolution, and experiencing a life of love and compassion. When we make healing an intentional part of daily living, we experience more directly the holistic interconnectedness of our physical body and the non-physical aspects of our lives like our emotions and the nature of our thinking. Healing bridges the gap between our physical bodies and our mental, emotional, and spiritual capacities.

Our experience of life is very different when healing is absent, ignored, or we are struggling to find the time and space for it. For many of us, our adult lives prioritize almost everything other than our own health and healing. The way we relate to our job responsibilities and our pursuit of money, our parenting, our obligations to school and grades, the seemingly endless "to do" lists—these things become so dominant in our lives that we often feel deeply out of balance, or we might be so entrenched in coping strategies that we don't even see how out of balance we are. When we become so hyper-focused on external demands, it is easy to feel overwhelmed. Before we know it, nurturing ourselves falls by the wayside, and we are left wondering why our bodies are in constant pain, why we experience so much distress, why we are frequently dissatisfied by our work, why we feel separate, lonely, and disconnected, and why our relationships are frequently unfulfilling.

If the primary focus of our lives is always on external demands, awareness of our internal emotional and spiritual needs often becomes dim; our internal needs recede into the background until we almost don't notice that we have them at all.

Many people believe that the circumstances of their lives dictate their actions. Things "just happen," and many of us believe that we simply don't have time or space in our lives to heal. We may feel victimized by our parenting obligations or because our jobs demand so much of our energy and attention. In our fast-paced world, we are so oriented toward *doing* that we think our choices are being made for us. Healing, however, is more related to how we are *being* than it is dependent on the actions we take. Because of our chronic busyness, we often neglect and lose access to different ways of being that allow for healing to take place in our lives. Healing reminds us that we are human beings, not human doers.

There are many tools and practices that facilitate intentional healing. Among them are trust, forgiveness, and compassion. When we are deeply connected to these energies—not merely as intellectual ideals or beliefs held in the mind—healing is more present in our lives. We are more available to the possibility and process of healing when we create and call forth trust, forgiveness, and compassion. These capacities exist on a vibrational level and, when accessed, their energetic frequency invites healing into all aspects of our lives. It isn't that trust or compassion are themselves healing per se (though they may be). They simply allow for healing because we are no longer exclusively preoccupied with the conditioned reactive story the mind creates about our experience; a story that may be impeding our openness to heal. The energetic frequencies of trust, compassion and forgiveness are pathways for us to get out of our head and into a space of much greater possibility for healing.

At its heart, healing provides us the capacity and space to perceive things in our lives—both in our external circumstances and our internal experiences—that we thought were concrete and impermeable, as fluid and changing. Healing is about reclaiming an awareness of life's essential wisdom. It requires a willingness to observe ourselves within our circumstances and notice the knee-jerk interpretations we make about those circumstances. Often times, we believe that we understand what life is communicating to us, but in actuality, we are responding to life based on our unconscious conditioning. Healing is our pathway to being with life as it is, without attachment to judgment.

Healing is not simply a rational process, nor is it dependent on how "smart" we are. If healing were primarily about intelligence, very intelligent people would be the best healers. Rather, healing requires a deep listening and understanding of those energies and patterns that preclude our connection to wholeness. Clearing blocked energy makes it easier for us to listen to and integrate the messages and wisdom of our bodies, which is an integral part of the healing process. Life is constantly communicating to us through our physical sensations, emotions, and thoughts. Having a better understanding of how life communicates with us in these ways is an integral part of the healing process.

Sometimes it might seem like healing demands that we have to give up what is important to us or what others expect of us. But healing is really about reclaiming an awareness of life's essential wisdom—the wisdom of remembering who we really are; the wisdom of allowing the power of love to take over our lives; and the wisdom of appreciating our interconnectedness with all parts of ourselves and others—leaving us with a deep sense of the sacredness of all of life.

When we finally choose to live a life that is connected, nurturing, and supported by healthy habits, it is very useful for us to learn about the context in which healing takes place and how we can have greater access to our innate capacity to heal ourselves. There are many qualities that we can all strive to cultivate in our lives that provide us with experiences we might call healing—experiences that have us feel more connected.

Healing can be the biggest gift we choose to give ourselves, as well as one of the most challenging to accept.

Healing Visualization

Center and Relax. Take a few deep breaths to let go of any tension in your body. Take as much time as you need to let your body and mind settle.

On a clean sheet of paper in your journal, write the word "Healing" at the top.

Write down five areas of your life in which you feel most connected, perhaps in your relationship to your life purpose, your family, your body, your relationship with the Nature, or with your significant other. What is it about these areas that has you feel so connected and fulfilled by them?

Then write down five areas of your life that you feel most disconnected, unresolved, or separated from. What is the opportunity for you if you any of these areas were healed? Do you know what you would have to do or who you would have to be to move forward in healing these areas?

Close your eyes, breathe deeply through your heart and allow yourself to sit in the space of this possibility for several minutes. After a few deep breaths, open your eyes and write down a few reflections on your process.

INTENTION AND EXPECTATION

"Do or do not; there is no try."

——YODA

One of the pillars of healing is having a clear intention of your purpose and your goal in life. A purpose is ongoing; it is the direction in which we are heading. A goal is concrete, measurable, and observable; it is finite and exists within a frame of time. Reorienting our lives within a context of intention, firmly rooted in a clear set of goals, allows us to be more aware of the ongoing healing presence that always exists within us. Because healing is so contingent on awareness, developing a clearer mind of what you intend and expect to experience is a vital part of healing. Similarly, uncovering and being aware of our buried negative thoughts and repetitive patterns that subvert our goals is important so that your positive intentions for healing can prevail.

For example, even if we say we'd like to get over our allergies, stabilize our blood sugar, lose weight, or whatever other health goals we might have, many of us unconsciously expect to fail at achieving these goals. Somewhere in our unconscious psyche is a conditioned narrative of expectation that assumes that what has been will always be; the allergies will never go away, the weight will never stay off, the stress will never be reduced. Our sense of possibility is compromised by our expectation and beliefs. It is important to understand that healing in this context—with this undercurrent of negative expectation—just isn't likely. We may experience temporary alleviation, we might lose weight for a time or improve our digestion, but in the vast majority of cases, the sheer force of our unconscious negative expectations will bring us right back to where we began. Healing is not about a temporary adjustment in circumstances; it is about a transformation of how we live our lives at a fundamental level. It is about reconnecting seemingly separate parts of ourselves with our innate wholeness and creating pathways for deeper levels of that connection.

Fundamentally, living life guided by our intentions creates a greater sense of choice. Often times, when we are faced with distracting symptoms, whether physical or emotional, our perceived sense of choice is diminished. When we are uncomfortable or in pain, our minds can become preoccupied by the story surrounding the symptoms—the circumstances that created them and the time line in which they occur. We begin to anticipate and judge and predict how the symptoms will play out. Before we know it, we are living in a world where the symptoms are happening to us and our experience of personal power all but disappears. However, when our intention is clear and we are unencumbered by negative repeating thought patterns that dictate our experience, we maintain our sense of choice—of co-creating our lives—even when we experience uncomfortable circumstances.

Living our lives from intention, rather than from conditioned patterns of thought, is a practice that can free us from painful identities and open us up to greater possibilities of healing. Intention requires a powerful commitment to move beyond ingrained habits of thinking and identification so that we can more fully embody our natural capacities as healers. As we make a practice of deepening our awareness of what's possible beyond our conditioned expectations, we are able to shift our focus and clarify what we positively intend for our lives. This practice frees us from being mechanically governed by the unconscious set of negative expectations that underpin much of our identities.

Healing Visualization:
Clarifying Your Intention to Heal

Make yourself comfortable. Imagine yourself laying peacefully in a meadow that feels warm and inviting. Lay down and feel your body totally relaxing, supported by the earth beneath you. Notice the clouds and the deep blue sky up above. Allow yourself to feel uplifted, inspired, and at peace here for however long you like.

After a few moments have passed, gently suggest to yourself the question, "What are my intentions for health and healing?" Hold the question lightly and notice what naturally arises, either in thought or feeling. If needed, gently repeat the question to yourself until your intentions become clear.

When you are ready, find a clean sheet in your journal and write "Healing Intentions" at the top. Make some notes from your visualization.

Write down your purpose for what you intend to heal. Where are you heading? What is it in service to? Then list the specific, measurable goals for your healing. When will you take action for each goal? What support do you need?

When it feels appropriate, share your commitments and intentions with someone you trust who can help hold you accountable for reaching your goals and will celebrate with you when you have accomplished them. Choose whether you would like to keep this list somewhere where you can reference it easily and be reminded of your purpose and your intention. Make a time in the next week to re-evaluate, clarify, and re-commit to your intentions.

THE MIND, BELIEFS, AND IDENTITIES

*"I must be willing to give up what I am in
order to become what I will be."*

—— ALBERT EINSTEIN

To understand what we unconsciously expect to happen, we have
to better understand how our mind works, because it is integral to
how we build and store our sense of identity in ways we don't often
recognize. For instance, while almost everyone has a desire to feel
healthy and fulfilled, many of us also argue for our physical and
emotional limitations. In the same breath, we will both declare our
desire to heal and rationalize why we can't, because many of us have
a closely held (unconscious) identity as someone who cannot heal.
Healing, then, must include a willingness to no longer be "right"
about what we think we cannot do and who we cannot be. When
we make excuses because of what we perceive are our limitations,
we are, in effect, choosing to stay in what we know, even in the
midst of our pain or discomfort. It's a paradox, but one we must
confront if we truly wish to bring healing into our lives.

Because most of our limitations are stored in the mind, we
can sometimes confuse our sense of self with very painful identities, such as someone who is—by definition—sick, overweight,
depressed, or incapable. There are countless ways we allow our
thoughts about ourselves to direct and influence who we take ourselves to be, rather than recognizing them as conditioned patterns
of thought that do not define our true nature.

Have you ever noticed that one of the first questions someone asks you when you first meet is, "So, what do you do"? Curious, isn't it? Of all the things you might want to know about someone, this is what we seek to find out first. Even more curious, perhaps, is that we have basically the same answer at the ready each time we are asked. This makes sense if you live in a culture where most people identify and value themselves by what they do. It's not too long in most conversations until we ask the next question: "Where are you from"? It is important to realize that a fundamental part of how we conceive of our lives is through what we do and where we've come from, and not just in terms of our profession or place of origin; our habitual actions and our experiential histories determine a great deal of how we understand who we are, how others characterize us, and how we characterize others. A story of who we are develops over time that we then exchange with one another as a way of explaining what is important to us. But is that really what we are? Is the most essential part of us the story we tell others about what we do and where we come from? Do we come to believe that story ourselves?

The identities that we develop over time help us navigate the world. We construct patterns of thought and systems of belief that help us make sense of what we encounter and what we experience. For most of us, however, this is an unconscious process, and we don't recognize how deeply attached we can become to our beliefs, especially those that help us reference who we are. If part of our deeply held belief system is that it is impossible or difficult for us to heal or that some things are unhealable, we will unconsciously go out of our way to make that belief correct.

This brings us back to the vital importance of awareness. Becoming aware of our negative beliefs and identities is a fundamental part of the healing process. If you can recognize that part of who you are *being*— as influenced by your belief system and identity—has an investment in keeping your identity as it is, then it's easy to see that healing requires a shift in identity, a shift in your state of being, and a release of those beliefs that are no longer serving your healing. As long as you focus exclusively on changing the outer world and the circumstances "out there"—including your physical symptoms—your healing process is incomplete. The patterns that continue to inform your experience—your thoughts, your beliefs, and who you take yourself to be—remain unchanged.

Begin cultivating an orientation to life as someone who naturally facilitates healing, someone for whom healing is a regular part of how you live. This may be unfamiliar territory for you, and it may require a shift in focus from the realm of doing to the realm of being. Most people don't consider themselves to be healers; healing, we believe, comes from an external source of authority, someone who "knows" what healing is and can give it to us. Many of us believe that healing is a rational process and that the body abides by a discrete linear set of universal laws. In that model, we don't need to "be" anyone different; we just need to acquire the right information, wait for the right time, and act accordingly in order to be healed. Healing, however, is not about waiting for the right time or the right circumstances. It is about who we are being now, in the present circumstances.

Coming to understand the interconnected and dynamic nature of our mind, body, and identity is a crucial part of seeing how our thoughts and attitude affect our capacity to heal. If our identity is for the most part caught up in unconscious negative beliefs about what is and is not possible for us, we will often feel disempowered in our ability to discover and welcome opportunities for healing into our lives. Bringing to light our negative beliefs and actively putting our commitment and intention into cultivating a deep relationship with our inherent ability to heal is one of the most transformative choices you may make in your journey of healing.

Healing Visualization:
Commit to Being a Healing Presence

Allow your body to relax and release any tension you may be holding. Breathe deeply and feel yourself returning to the present moment. Take as much time as you need to feel centered and present.

In your journal, write a letter to yourself beginning with "Dear [your name]". Then, write yourself caring, loving words from your heart about what you yearn to heal and what conflicts you feel may be blocking you.

Conclude your letter with a commitment to live your life as a healing presence, both for yourself and those with whom you share this life.

EMOTIONS

"The best and most beautiful things in the world cannot be seen or even touched. They must be felt with the heart."

— HELEN KELLER

Healing demands more than an intellectual questioning of "why" something happened in a past or present moment. It requires both identifying and removing the energetic blocks that we carry within us. Giving ourselves permission to experience the depth of our feelings allows us to be more in tune with important steps of healing.

An inherent distinction between human beings and all other animals is that we have the opportunity to experience and identify an enormous range and variety of emotions. The purpose of our feelings is for us to learn how to experience them without attachment or judgment. However, it is challenging for most of us to experience what we judge to be negative, bad, wrong, or evil emotions. When we view emotions in a dichotomy of good and bad, it may seem counterintuitive for us to intentionally allow for experiences that we perceive to be only negative.

When we don't live in a context where our emotions are valuable and welcome, many of us will try to think our way through our experience instead. While profound intellectual insights can be very rewarding, our lives as human beings are not limited to processes of the mind. Life is meant to be experienced fully, and our emotions highlight the richness and breadth of what life has to offer.

When we diminish, stifle, or ignore our emotions, giving preference instead to the intellectual or the rational, we shut off access to one of the fundamental elements of what makes us human.

Most of us grow up in environments where the primary social and cultural context teaches us that some emotions are good and some emotions are bad. As children, we are often told that our expressions of emotion will not be tolerated. We witness our parents, siblings, and community reflexively stifling their own emotional experiences. How we perceive and relate to emotional expression is often deeply conditioned, and without even thinking about it, we develop categories in our mind for emotions that are "good" and emotions that are "bad." This moral framework compels us to seek "positive" emotional experiences while avoiding "negative" emotional experiences throughout our lives at almost any cost. Functionally, this can pose enormous challenges for us if it means we constantly live in opposition with the reality of our lives.

Anger is anger. Fear is fear. Feelings themselves are never the problem, although we often view them as such. When we add our judgments to our feeling experience, the expression of the feeling can become distorted as we perceive them through the filter of our judgment and expectation. Then, "negative" emotions cease to have value for us, because our sole purpose becomes escaping or changing the experience. It becomes enormously challenging to skillfully identify what exactly it is we are feeling when we believe it could be interpreted as evidence that something is wrong with us. If we could identify clearly what and how we are feeling, we might be more able to learn effective ways of expressing our feelings. If we learn effective skills to express our feelings, we might be able to investigate ways of releasing the energy of what we are experiencing.

Many of us have substantial amounts of conditioning that prohibits us from clearly or authentically expressing our feelings. We have grown up in families where we heard frequent injunctions like "stop crying or I'll give you something to cry about," "Why are you angry? You have no right to be angry!" or "Stop being so sensitive!"

On the other hand, others of us come from backgrounds that give us license to passionately express any feeling, at any time, under any circumstance. Neither extreme facilitates a grounded healing process. If someone develops a habit of suppressing their anger—either because they are told it is unacceptable to be angry or they simply don't know how to express it authentically—the suppression of that energy can build over time. Not only might it make them more sensitive and intolerant of situations where anger arises in the future, but it may also be expressed physically as colitis, cancer, or other chronic physical symptoms. Constantly suppressing our emotional experience takes enormous energy and awareness, which can lead to us feeling chronically tired, overwhelmed, and preoccupied. This process of expressing our emotional feelings through physical symptoms is called somatization, and is common for those who are unaware of their emotional feelings.

Giving ourselves permission to experience and express the truth of our emotional landscape doesn't mean that we will never feel pain. Our assessment, however, of the pain will be fundamentally different. The traumas that confront us in life are both big and small, but it is how we meet them that determines our experience. Unfortunately, the approach of ignore-and-suppress doesn't clear energy, and because painful energetic patterns get embedded into our body when we aren't clearing them, we set ourselves up to deal with uncomfortable and painful feelings the same way in the future, over and over again.

One of the keys to healing is not just expressing what we feel but also learning how to release the energy of the feeling so that we don't carry the energy around with us. When you don't fully express and release feelings, the energy from them is stored in the tissues and structure of the body and in the identity structures of the mind. One might refer to them as "non-experienced experiences," and we live our lives as if they don't have any power or they don't exist at all. In truth, non-experienced experiences have profound influence over how we think, feel, and act. However, because we don't consciously bring them into our awareness for processing and release, they can insidiously show up as recurring blocks to our sense of freedom, enjoyment of life, and our peace of mind. Both the energy of non-experienced experiences and the repetitive patterns they produce continue to shape us until the energy is cleared.

Healing is about getting complete with our non-experienced experiences and releasing the energy that may be causing us continued physical and emotional distress. When you commit to healing, it requires that you practice awareness so that you become familiar with the patterns that non-experienced experiences create in your life. When we develop skillful awareness, the process of healing becomes revelatory, exciting, and transformative, as the stagnant energies in our body are released and we regain our innate sense of freedom and peace.

Healing Visualization:
Healing Our Heart

Imagine yourself inside a large translucent blue bubble big enough for you to step inside. The bubble has a lounge chair with cushions and more than enough oxygen, making it easy to feel comfortable, safe, and protected. Let yourself relax inside the bubble, feeling the soft blue light gently warming your skin. Being in the bubble, you can let any tension ease out of your body.

When the time feels right, allow yourself to recall a time when you were hurt, angry, or afraid. Allow the memory to be clear in your mind, noting the time, place, and circumstances of the moment. What happened to have you feel this way? Who was with you? What did you feel? Notice where in your body your feelings are located. Allow yourself to acknowledge and accept any mental reactions, feelings, or physical sensations that arise regarding the circumstance. Remember, you are in the protective environment of the blue bubble. Bring your awareness back to breathing in the blue healing light as you visualize.

See yourself writing this all down in detail. When you have completely written down the memory in your mind, imagine a strong fire burning in a fireplace. Place the piece of paper with your memory into the fire and watch the smoke waft up toward the sky. Allow the burning of the paper to cleanse you of any residual emotional energy related to the memory.

This may be a substantial catharsis for you, so be sure to give yourself as much space as you need to fully allow the energy to be released from your body. Write down any reflections, thoughts, or feelings you have about the experience in your journal.

Consider repeating this visualization once a week for the next month, following the steps closely each time.

OBSERVING ENERGY AND PATTERNS

"If you want to find the secrets of the universe, think in terms of energy, frequency and vibration."

— Nikola Tesla

One of the ways we can deepen our sense of awareness is by coming into contact with the subtle energies of our body. Our bodies are made of energy, and quantum physics tells us that the very root of all matter in the universe is energy. For most of us, however, we do not perceive energy when we look out into the world; we see solid physical objects. We see our bodies, structures, nature, people and so forth. The physical world, for the most part, dominates our perception, but there is so much more about our lives than what we see.

Many of us conceptually understand that everything is energy. We have either studied it in physics, read about it in an esoteric text, or discussed chi and meridians with our acupuncturists. Many paradigms for understanding energy as a concept have appeared throughout the ages, and cultivating an awareness and relationship to the energies in your body is transformative. Understanding something conceptually, however, is very different than having an experiential awareness of how it shows up in your own life. Ultimately, the words we use to describe something are not as important as the direct experience itself.

We can directly see how energy works in our lives by learning to observe our experience without judgment. Developing the ability to observe our experience without judgment is a profoundly valuable skill that opens up our capacity for healing. Most people, however, confuse observation with interpretation. The two things happen almost simultaneously with one another. The eye sees and the mind interprets; the body feels and the mind interprets. Experience-and-interpret over and over again. We rarely take the opportunity to just be with things as they are in their natural state. We have difficulty separating the experiences we perceive with the meaning—often in the form of a judgment—that accompanies the observation. And this is exactly where we want to begin: noticing that we unconsciously and reflexively assign meaning and judgment to our experience. For most of us, we only see reality through the interpretive lens of the mind, though we think we perceive the world objectively.

One of the practices offered during the LOVE YOUR BODY programs came to be known as the Mirror Process. At night before bed or early in the morning after you wake up, you stand in front of a full length mirror naked and simply observe your physical body noticing the commentary from your mind. Most people have so many unconscious or negative assessments about their physical appearance that simply *being* with their body without letting the thoughts spiral can be very challenging. The opportunity for transformation, however, is enormous. If we can see that how we conceive of ourselves is often nothing more than a story produced over years, there is the space suddenly to discover who we truly are in this moment.

A woman who had taken the program a number of times had such a breakthrough with the mirror process that she put a mirror on the ceiling in her bathroom so that when she took a bath each night, she could look at her body and feel all of the love and acknowledgement for how wonderful it was that she had a body to honor, respect, and use in this life to connect with other people.

Learning to see ourselves without the cloud of judgment from our thoughts can be life-changing. It isn't that we force ourselves to think better, more positive thoughts, but by observing ourselves without judgment we are able to come into deeper connection with who we truly are. Transformation doesn't occur through coercion; it occurs through awareness.

Something that we come to notice when we are able to observe our experience more intimately is that much of our physical and emotional experience occurs in patterns. Energy develops into patterns easily, both in its physical form and in its subtle forms. Most of us can remember visiting our pediatrician when we were little and having the doctor knock on the side of our knee with a small rubber hammer, prompting us to give a little kick reflexively. This is the patellar ligament reflex, and it is works by stimulating the nerve that causes the muscles in your leg to kick. If you were to knock on your patellar with the little hammer every hour for a month, your leg would be so trained that it would continue giving a little kick every hour for the rest of your life, even without the stimulus of the hammer.

Habitual reactions train patterns into our lives, physically and emotionally. Some of these patterns are intentional and beneficial, while others are unconscious and limiting. For competitive and professional athletes, developing a "muscle memory" for the movements that make up their sport is of the utmost importance. By repeating the motions over and over again, we both condition and strengthen the muscles that perform the movement and we pattern the neural pathways in our brain that trigger the movement. As we practice over time, the muscle fibers "remember" the movement and can perform it more quickly and more reliably when we fire the neural command.

To get that level of training and reflexivity, we need to practice. The act of practice requires a conscious intention for us to stimulate the reaction we are trying to develop. Athletes spend hours and hours meticulously correcting their form; the pitcher's arm must be at the perfect angle with the perfect velocity to execute the pitch correctly; the stroke of the tennis player's follow-through must be just so in order to send the ball to the exact position on the other side of the court. Consciously conditioning our bodies during practice is intended to build such instantaneous access to the movement that we don't have to think about the form during competition; it just occurs naturally. We have programmed our muscles and our nervous system to execute on command when we need them to, allowing us to focus on other things in the moment.

The subtle energies in our body—thoughts, feelings, sensations—can be similarly patterned, though we are often unconscious of the process we go through to create these patterns. We come into contact with energy and stimulus from the outside world all the time. Every person we meet, every conversation we have, everything we read, everything we watch on TV- energetic exchanges are happening every second of our lives, but we often lack the awareness to see the relationship between those exchanges and the thoughts, feelings, and sensations we experience. We assume that thoughts and feelings arise spontaneously and objectively according to each circumstance, rather than as a result of energetic patterns we hold in our body.

Because the energetic component of our experience is so infrequently discussed in our culture, many of us are unaware that we hold energetic patterns that specifically hinder our healing process. The first step to releasing these patterns is developing the capacity to simply observe our experience without adding a mental assessment or judgment to the experience. This allows us to observe how our thoughts and feelings are wired, how they've been programmed throughout our lives. For some, it is radical to even consider that we might be able to observe our mental and emotional conditioning and then be able to consciously change it. Releasing the energetic patterns in our body that drive our unconscious emotional and mental reactions is a fundamental aspect of healing.

THE CONDITIONED MIND

The conditioned mind refers to the mechanistic, reactionary aspect of our lives. It is an unconscious part of our mind, programmed by our past experiences, our beliefs, and our environment. The conditioned mind has us perceive and respond to the world in a way that may not be in alignment with our deepest sense of self or our deepest values. When we are living from our conditioned mind, we are not living spontaneously, and we may feel an absence of freedom and choice.

And yet, this is not a mental process; if anything it is a capacity of our deepest state of being. Understanding that we have conditioning that might not serve us does not in and of itself release us from the conditioning. How many of us know someone in our lives who can tell you exactly what triggers them and exactly how they will react, yet still react that way on a regular basis? Someone who knows they are an alcoholic is not cured just by acknowledging their addiction. Knowing our patterns doesn't undo them. We must undertake an intentional, conscious process to release the energy embedded within us that runs the pattern and then consciously replace it with a process that serves our wholeness. While understanding and gaining insight can be useful, reprogramming our conditioned mind requires us to access a place that is beyond our usual rational, discursive, and logical processes.

We can do this in a number of ways, but as we discussed earlier, having a clear intention is of paramount importance. Being able to discern between observation and interpretation is also important. Certain capacities of the spirit—trust, forgiveness, and compassion, for instance—can be cultivated to aid us in releasing energy that is trapped in the body. When we stand firmly in our commitment to our own healing, doorways and possibilities open up to us almost immediately. When we consciously choose to observe our experience without judgment and begin re-patterning our energetic responses, we are no longer as susceptible to being taken over by emotions. Energy in our body may arise in the form of emotion, but we are no longer victims of reactive negative assessments about our experience. For most people, this is a radical change from the knee-jerk cycle of reactivity that most of us have come to expect.

CASE HISTORY
Using Mindfulness to Heal Tammy's Unhealthy Patterns

Tammy came to see me after a double mastectomy and reconstructive surgery. She had taken Tamoxafin for her breast cancer, felt extremely run down, and wanted to recover the physical energy to which she was accustomed. Like many of my clients, she was interested in detoxing the drugs and chemical residue from her body, so I suggested a food plan specific to her needs. Using fresh organic foods, medical protein powders, and herbs, we would support her body to clear the toxins that were not being eliminated by the normal routes of elimination.

I saw Tammy every few weeks to tweak and adjust the program; the stress her body had endured was severe and required a multi-level approach. In two months, Tammy said she was feeling terrific. She traveled to Europe for three weeks and returned feeling like her physical results were sustaining very well. When she came to see me for her follow up, she looked great, but something about her attitude caught my attention. Now that her energy had returned, Tammy was ready to return to life as usual, which for her was a fast-paced schedule of constant activity. At 60, she was deeply invested in her work life and considered herself an overachiever. She resented the time that an ongoing program of relaxation, healthy eating, and self-care would take.

There is no doubt that Tammy is a courageous woman. Even after a painful bout with cancer, losing two breasts, and going through reconstructive surgery, she still loved her adrenalin-filled life and still took on more than any average five people combined. With each success and accomplishment at work, she was driven to go farther and take on more. The work would mount, the rewards would follow, and she would feed off of the rush. Her lack of intimacy with her husband and an absent sex life was a small price, in her estimation, to pay.

I invited Tammy to work with me and allow me to coach her about space. I promised her she could continue to feel great about her drive at work while still fulfilling her commitment to healing. Her healing did not mean she had to stop loving her work or stop being an overachiever, but it did require that she release some of the patterns that were no longer serving her optimal wellness and posed the risk of undermining her health in the future.

I offered Tammy a distinction between nourishing and nurturing. Nourishing means giving the body the foods it needs to work well. Everyone's body is different. We all have specific needs that change and evolve. Knowing how to listen to our body and make adjustments to what we eat and what supplements we use takes practice, patience, and a willingness to be flexible. Knowing how to nourish yourself is related to optimal health.

Nurturing is what allows you to connect to your heart and create space in your life. The healing opportunity from Tammy's breast cancer was offering her a new possibility for how she could relate to wellness, beyond deriving satisfaction from the mind's sense of success and the constant pursuit of ambition.

As I coached Tammy on presence and mindfulness, she revealed that in her family growing up, there was no space for anyone to ever get sick. It was a sign of weakness to be resisted and fought at all costs. Food, similarly, was an unfortunate necessity, and the sooner the meal was over the better. Because these patterns were unresolved, she resisted continuing to follow a healthy food plan that would support her ongoing optimal health. These ways of relating to food and health were deeply conditioned into Tammy's ways of thinking, and I asked her to consider that it might be necessary to release the energy from these patterns that were inhibiting her from fully healing from the breast cancer. What if food was a good source of nourishment that she could take joy in? What if sickness was not weakness, but information from the body, an opportunity to heal and learn something quite profound?

Visualization:
Releasing Energetic Patterns

Imagine yourself lying comfortably on a beach. The sun glistens on the water and gulls call playfully in the distance. The water washes gently onto the shore and you feel your whole body relaxing.

Feel the lightness of your whole being, as if the sunshine and your physical body had no boundary between them. Picture yourself glowing as if made of pure light energy. The contour of your body is wreathed in light and you feel yourself beginning to float up, leaving your physical body behind. Notice the lightness of your being as you look back toward your body, comfortably resting on the beach. Allow yourself to feel the freedom of being. As you look back on your body below, notice if you can be with the physical aspect of your life without judging or assessing. Just be. Continue to observe your physical body hovering over it in your suit of illuminated light for several minutes.

Come down to be closer to your physical body, as you continue connecting with your body of light and kneel in silence near the top of your head. Gently put your hands of light on the head of your physical body and give yourself permission to release any tension or negative patterns that your physical body holds. As you send this healing energy to yourself, breathe deeply. Can you feel a lightness or relief in your heart? If you feel comfortable, take the glowing right hand of light on your physical heart and your glowing left hand under your physical neck. Stay with this connection in your imagination for a few minutes. Keep breathing calmly and deeply. Feel the energy of your light body flowing into your physical body.

If any feelings or emotions arise, simply allow them to be with you as you continue the process of giving yourself healing energy. Continue to offer this silent prayer, giving yourself permission to let go of the energy that blocks your complete healing. When the time feels right, feel your light body and physical body begin to merge once again. As the two become one, and you are fully back, present in your physical body, notice the place within you where the peace and beauty of the beach always lives.

When you feel that the visualization is complete, take out your journal and write down any thoughts, feelings, or insights about what you've just experienced. Repeat this process again each week for the next month, allowing the freedom and release you experience to deepen each time.

TRUST

"The goal of life is to make your heartbeat match the beat of the universe, to match your nature with nature."

—JOSEPH CAMPBELL

"...teach us to take our hearts and look them in the face, however difficult it may be."

—DOROTHY SAYERS

Innate to being in a human body is the capacity to heal. When we get a scrape, the body knows how to repair the skin; when we catch a cold, the immune system boosts white blood cells to remove the pathogen; the cells in our body are in a constant state of birth, decay, death, and regeneration. Healing is a fundamental part of being alive, and when we are in relationship with the innate wisdom of the body to heal itself, our trust deepens, and with it, our experience of peace.

Living in deep connection with this innate capacity for healing is itself a transformative process. To trust this capacity—to truly trust yourself—is to locate your identity outside of the mind's story of who you are. Trust invites an entirely different quality of being and focus into your life, one that is fundamentally welcoming to the healing process. When trust is present, the mind that seeks to know right answers settles; the personality trying to control the circumstances of life lets go. Trust is about letting go of our preconceived notions of how life should be, so that we can really be present in the moment, rather than ruminating over the past, or worrying about the future.

Healing is not only an automated process that the body carries out unconsciously or that just happens in life. True, healing can happen spontaneously, and does for many of us at different times. Life by itself can be very healing without our knowing or being involved. However, when we intentionally connect to those facets of our being that generate healing, we can bring it more fully into our lives.

Most of us, however, have a difficult time connecting to trust because we are overcome by fear. There is a Tibetan Buddhist saying: "Believing doubt is the slayer of spirit." Fear can be an overwhelming challenge that blocks our access to the possibility of healing. Fear is one of those aspects of life that most of us spend incredible amounts of time avoiding or developing coping strategies to deal with. As part of the process of having greater connection to trust, we may need to heal our relationship with fear; not get over it or beyond it necessarily, but shift the context in which fear shows up in our lives so that we can meet it with grace and dignity, and learn from its power. The beginning of trust is the sense of its necessity for healing.

Healing fear, however, can be elusive and tricky, because we have so many negative judgments about fear when we begin to experience it. Negative judgment is a way of resisting fear, which has the effect of actually solidifying it in our experience, not relieving it. Observing the assessments we make about fear when it arises is often necessary to getting some space from the intensity of the fear. It can be as if the emotion hijacks us and we are no longer able to observe ourselves. We become so overidentified with the experience of overwhelm that we cannot consider much else. While it may seem counterintuitive, accepting the presence of fear—rather than resisting it—is the fundamental step to opening up access to trust, and, therefore, bringing healing into our lives more intentionally.

Most people defer to outer authorities to confirm what is rational to trust or not. In other words, they externalize their sense of trust, rather than locating it deep within themselves. The kind of trust that is premised on reasonable evidence is actually not a very deep or powerful kind of trust. The circumstances of the external world are in constant flux, and if our connection to trust relies on the external, it too is subject to vacillation and change. Our trust then has no real integrity because it is not located inside of us. We can all cultivate and learn how to listen to that place of trust that abides within us and offers us the experience of being a healing presence.

*

I love the story about the hiker walking along a mountain path.

While enjoying the beautiful scenery, the hiker suddenly trips, falls off the path, and barely manages to grab hold of a branch protruding from the side of the mountain. Holding on for dear life, the hiker begins shouting, "Help! Help! Is anyone up there?" Down below, there is only the abyss. Above, the edge of the path is way beyond reach. "Help, help, can anyone hear me?" the hiker desperately yells again.

A calm, confident and clear voice from above suddenly responds, "It is okay. You are okay." The hiker is relieved beyond imagination and says, "Great! Who is that?" The resonant source voice replies, "This is God."

"Oh, God! How great that you're here! Tell me what to do." The hiker says, delighted that someone has come to the rescue.

God lovingly says: "Let go."

Without much hesitation, the hiker looks up and shouts, "Is anyone else up there?"

After a bit of time, with no other options, the hiker lets go, only to land on a small platform of rock jutting out from the side of the mountain that was impossible to see. Sometimes we need to let go before we can see our way.

Visualization: Leaning into Trust

Take a few minutes to relax, center, and connect to your goals and intentions for healing. Allow your commitment to be a healing presence in the world to come into the center of your experience. When you feel connected to your purpose, find a clean sheet in your journal and write down the two following lists

List 1 : Who are the people in your life who taught you how to trust? This list can contain real people or a character from literature or history who you find inspiring. Next to each person's name be specific about how you learned trust from this person.

List 2 : Who are the people who encouraged your skepticism, your cynicism, and instilled in you a belief that there are many things in this world that you cannot trust. Be specific about what you learned from this person.

Take a moment to reflect on these lists. How do they continue to influence and bare an impact on your life today?

Next, on another clean page write a love letter to those parts of you that live in fear. Using the following questions to guide you, begin with "Dear Fearful (your name)]

How you have learned to distrust people, the world, and yourself ?

What beliefs and actions are directly related to how you do not trust? Be specific.

How do you act that others might call controlling?

How do you trust yourself in spite of fearful situations? How do you show that you trust others?

What are you committed to heal about the fear and trust in your life?

After you spend some time with these questions, write down any thoughts, feelings, and insights you have about what generates and sustains trust as well as what inhibits trust in your life. Return to these questions regularly as a part of your ongoing practice in developing trust in service to your healing.

FORGIVENESS AND COMPASSION

*"Real forgiveness is giving up the hope that
the past could have been any different."*
— MICHAEL BECKWITH

*"Our sorrows and wounds are healed only
when we touch them with compassion."*
— THE BUDDHA

At the root of transformational healing is a connection to love and a sense of wholeness that is fundamental to who we are. Without love, we cannot fully heal, because healing does not come from a state of separation, and we remain disconnected when love is absent from our lives. An injury might improve or some disease symptoms might abate, but without love, we cannot be connected to our wholeness. In order for us to embody that connection fully, we must have forgiveness and compassion for ourselves as well as for the circumstances of our lives.

First, it may be useful to make a distinction about what forgiveness is and what it isn't. Many people assume that forgiveness exists for the sake of another, perhaps for someone who has hurt or offended you. You may contemplate whether they are worthy of forgiveness, whether they have repented sufficiently, and, on that basis determine whether or not you will forgive. This approach to forgiveness does not necessarily take into consideration how you will restore your own sense of connection and deepen the presence of love in your life that has been eroded by the insult.

True forgiveness is, in fact, about you. To truly forgive is restorative and reconnecting. Forgiveness is an affirmation of our dedication to be a healing presence in the world, for ourselves, and for others. Moments of conflict and hurt can sometimes become about power and manipulation, rather than healing. If someone has hurt you, you may feel that the question of forgiveness is about how you can then control them or exact some retribution before you decide to forgive. If you are very hurt, perhaps the way you feel safe again is by excluding them from your life in order to regain some semblance of security. True forgiveness—the kind that restores you to your sense of wholeness, regardless of the external circumstances—has no preconditions.

There is no obligation to forgive. Choosing to forgive or not to forgive has different consequences. The benefits of not forgiving are, in some ways, very enticing. We get to stay right, we avoid being dominated, and we are not confronted with being responsible for our experience. The cost of not forgiving is simple, but grave. We lose some of our capacity to love and feel loved—intimacy is beyond us. We close ourselves off and diminish our capacity for connection. Without connection and love, however, there is no healing. With connection and love, on the other hand, we do not maintain a position of righteousness or judgment.

So, how do we connect to forgiveness when the intensity of hurting and indignation can sometimes overwhelm our experience? Depending on the circumstances, forgiveness can seem like a difficult or even impossible task, and cutting ourselves off or isolating the antagonist might feel like the only thing we can do to get some reprieve from our suffering. Forgiveness may not mean instantaneous dissolution of all negative feelings; it simply begins with the firm commitment and declaration to heal the disconnection that was created.

Fundamental to opening up the possibility for forgiveness is compassion. Compassion is what allows things to be as they are with deep love and intimacy and without judgment. It is not an action we take, but a space we hold that allows connection to be present even in the midst of discomfort and conflict. As His Holiness the Dalai Lama says, "If you want others to be happy, practice compassion. If you want to be happy, practice compassion."

And compassion most certainly is a practice. It is the ongoing invitation to be with your experience—and the experience of others—just as it is, outside the judging mind. It is a practice that we develop for ourselves and for the sake of others. In its presence, true forgiveness is the natural progression of our journey to healing.

Now, to be clear, forgiveness is not about ignoring injustice; it is not denial. However, it is not necessary for conditions of reparation to be made before we release the toxic energy of hate and judgment from within us by forgiving. Forgiveness is a gift we give ourselves—not necessarily a gift we only give to others—because it facilitates being present to our own wholeness, and when we are whole, we are healed. When we are experiencing our wholeness, we are then a healing presence in the world and are capable of serving others in deep and meaningful ways.

Forgiveness is a transformative process because it can touch every aspect of our lives that is unhealed, especially those areas we thought could not be healed. It heals traumas in our past; it heals the fear of a terrifying diagnosis; it heals the harsh words shared with a loved one. Forgiveness also invites us to atone for our own transgressions, especially those we have perpetrated against ourselves. Forgiveness is a process of completion. It is what allows unresolved toxic energies in the body to be released, which may have been inhibiting our connection to wholeness. The effects of true, deep forgiveness are instantaneous: our hearts open, tension releases from the body, and, most importantly, the opportunity to hold a much bigger space of healing and possibility in our life comes into being. Forgiveness is the key to freedom.

While our personal relationships will often provide challenges for our practice of forgiveness, it may be most difficult to forgive ourselves. Perhaps there was a period of time when we did not treat our physical body with the respect it deserved. Perhaps we let our anger get the better of us and hurt someone we cared for. A deep commitment to restoring our sense of wholeness comes about when we sincerely begin to forgive ourselves and atone for our own transgressions.

Healing Process:
Connecting to Forgiveness and Compassion

Write your answers to the following three exercises in your healing notebook. In either exercise just write whatever comes to you in response to the prompts, without analyzing what you write. These exercises are intended to access energy that lives in your body without any analysis or judgment from your mind.

Exercise 1:

- Think of someone you have not forgiven, someone for whom you still hold resentment.
- Think about what you would receive by forgiving them.
- Think about someone who has not forgiven you.
- Think about the effect it has on you knowing that you haven't been forgiven.

Take a few moments and write down the sensations in your body and listen to the feelings that arise when you reflect on these experiences. It isn't necessary to spend any time assessing or judging the circumstances of the experience. Simply stay with the felt sense of it.

Then, connect to that part of you that has a deep commitment to be a healing presence in the world. What or who would you need to forgive in order to more deeply embody that commitment? What atonement might you make that would anchor this commitment?

Make some notes that you can refer to that will help remind you of your commitment to heal and forgive.

Exercise 2:

On a new page, answer the following questions with whatever comes to mind most easily.

In your life, what have you done to yourself—to your body—for which you can forgive yourself?

What have you avoided or not done for yourself—for your body—for which you can forgive yourself?

Who has done something to you who you now forgive?

Who has not done something for you that you are now able to forgive?

Exercise 3:

For three minutes every day for one month, write the phrase: "I release, forgive, and bless [fill in the blank of someone's name. Could be your own.]

Remember, this is not a thinking process. Just allow your pen to write without mentally editorializing.

Visualizing Compassion

Relax and center yourself by focusing on the breath naturally coming in and out of the body. Allow any tension you may be holding to gradually and completely slip away.

Allow yourself to feel the presence of a holy person. This could be Jesus, the Buddha, Gandhi, Martin Luther King Jr., the Dalai Lama, or anyone you know personally in your life who has touched you in a spiritual way. Allow the loving energy of this being to embrace you and allow their loving energy to be present with you. Feel yourself anticipating and listening to the loving wisdom this being has come to offer you.

After a few moments of being silent, ask them the following questions one by one. Listen with the subtle knowing of your heart until the answer becomes clear:

- What is compassion ?
- How can you be more compassionate ?
- What specific practices can deepen my compassion for myself?

When you feel you have received a clear response, write in your journal to remind you of what you have learned from this teacher.

Repeat this as often as you wish with as many different wise beings as you like, taking the time each time to center, relax, and listen from your heart.

EMBRACING DEATH

"It is better to spend one day contemplating the birth and death of all things than a hundred years never contemplating beginnings and endings."

—— The Buddha

Is it possible that the whole purpose of life is to prepare yourself to die with dignity—that the relationships you develop over the course of your lifetime, the lessons you learn, and the challenges you confront are all meant to carry you forward, such that when the time comes for you to leave your physical body, you are complete, resolved, and at peace? Imagine for a moment that when your time comes, all of your affairs are in order, all of your relationships, past and present, are complete and without regret, and you have a deep and abiding sense of readiness for whatever comes next.

To die with dignity is to have lived life as a spiritual being having a physical experience. The physical body that has carried you through this lifetime may pass away, but for the core of who you are—your spirit—death is but a transition, a natural part of the life process. Form changing form. The process of dying does not contradict healing; it is a fundamental part of healing.

To approach death in this way, we must free ourselves from the notions we carry around in our mind about what death is. Death, many believe, is tragic, terrible, and to be avoided at all cost. Most of our ideas about death are caught up in profound fear because we do not know what happens after our physical body is no longer carrying us. The healing process in life is about reconnecting to our wholeness and shifting our identity away from the repetitive patterns of mind that keep us separate. When healing reconnects us with our own sense of spirit in a deep and meaningful way, our understanding of death fundamentally changes– it becomes a marker of transition, rather than a marker of ending.

Living life as a spiritual being is a sacred process. It is the root from whence we derive our commitment to be a healing presence in the world. Including death as a natural part of that commitment can be both confronting and transformative. Much of our culture sanitizes death as a way of staying distant from it. We numb ourselves by disconnecting from emotion, we retreat, or we let the bureaucracy of hospitals and institutions "manage" the process for us. We do this because we do not have a context that includes death as a part of life. We are not intentional about how we approach dying.

True, in some ways death is about loss. Our body passes away. The identity with a life we thought belonged to us passes away. The other way to look at death, however, is about deeply connecting with the essential nature of who you are. In a broad sense, healing arises out of a deep trust that the magnificence of your being is whole, complete, and without imperfection. Healing is about acceptance of what we are—not necessarily the acceptance of what appears to be or the meaning we ascribe to what we perceive; it is our re-union with what is real and actual about our lives. This kind of healing prepares us for dying with deep trust, connection, and compassion, without resistance.

In many instances, however, we are confronted with death or the prospect of dying before we believe our healing process is complete. No one can anticipate when their time will come. If you have been engaged in a deep and committed healing process for some time, you have more than likely cultivated a relationship with letting go of attachment. Death, ultimately is about freedom.

The process of letting go before we die offers us the opportunity to be truly free—free from the bondage of the ego mind, free from a lifetime of closely held beliefs and stories about what was or should have been. When we become very intimate with the dying process, everything about our lives gets put into a very different perspective. Death, like all things, takes place in the present moment. The more intimate we can be with this moment, the more freedom, connection, and love we will experience as our spirit transitions out of the physical world.

The most important to thing to realize about death is that it is always already happening. Each of us have been dying since the moment we were born. Living a life that includes death as an integral part of living enables us to be connected to the present, free of attachment to what comes and goes as our life journey continues.

Visualization:
Embracing Dying

Take a few moments to notice your breathing and begin allowing your body to relax. Any tension in your physical body, any emotions you may be experiencing—are all allowed to melt away. Inhale naturally as you bring a sense of calm and peace into your being.

When you feel centered, begin to imagine you are kneeling at a gravesite. As you read the headstone, you realize that this is where your physical body was commemorated after your death.

Recall the moments of your dying process that preceded your last physical breath.

See the people surrounding you who came to share space and remembrance with you as you made your transition, celebrating the enormous contribution you made to their lives.

Allow yourself to connect to your courage, trust, compassion, and the appreciation you feel for all the blessings you experienced during your time on earth. Take a few moments and allow yourself to fully feel the depth of how profoundly you allowed yourself to let go of your physical body with dignity. Give yourself time to remember all the different emotions you went through as you heard the call that it was your time to let go of your physical life.

Then, allow yourself to remember how it was to let go of your body as your breath left you. Give yourself permission to fully experience your personal process of dying. Take as much time as you need to be fully present with how death and dying was for you.

When it feels right, bring yourself back into your physical body. Feel the breath moving in and out of your lungs. Feel your own heartbeat. Come back and be fully present in your body in the room you're in now.

Then, in your healing journal, write down anything you noticed about your dying experience. What surprised you? What did you feel?

Take a few moments and write about what dying with dignity means to you. Having gone through the experience in your imagination, how would you have it be different in the future? What changes would you need to make—in being or in action—that would prepare you for the moment when you're called to let go.

Return to this exercise as an open exploration and investigation into your relationship with how to live and die with dignity.

Afterword

Dedication to a life of health and healing requires an ongoing practice of open-mindedness. The most profound transformations occur when we step out of the familiar and into the unknown; when our sense of expectation is overcome by the clarity of our awareness and something new spontaneously comes into being. This practice, of course, has implications way beyond our personal lives. What kind of world would we have for our children, for instance, if, as adults, we cherished and lived from values that encouraged health and healing? What would our world look like? If we answered these questions from the familiar conditioned patterns of mind, many of us might not even consider such a possibility. The weight of our expectation—our beliefs about society, the economy, the trajectory of the human family—might undermine our sense of what's possible. When we have no sense of what's possible, we are not really available for anything revolutionary. For truly transformative healing to take place in our lives, we must be willing to fully step outside of what we know in order to discover new possibilities.

When we clearly recognize the interrelated aspects that make up our individual lives—the systems within our physical body, our emotions, our spirit, and our mind—we may see that none of these things are actually separate or distinct entities. Rather, they are more like descriptions of phenomena within experience that inform how we understand existence. It is only one step further from this understanding to seeing the interrelatedness of all life. Consider for a moment the implications of living on a single planet with a finite set of resources. Finite freshwater, finite arable land, and, at the same time, a growing population that faces heretofore unimagined social stratification. At this moment in history, now more than ever, human beings are being forced to confront their place in the web of life and our role as a collective on Earth.

When we truly have a deep commitment to our own healing, we will recognize the origin of this commitment comes from beyond ourselves as individuals and our personal desire to heal. True healing is not exclusively for the purpose of you alone. Our inherent connection to one another, to the planet, and to all life means that our deep commitment to healing is actually in service to the cosmos. Personal healing is a gateway for awareness to recognize your fundamental connectedness with the universe. This will sound like a remote esoteric concept unless you are in deep connection with your purpose, aware, awake, and taking actions that are congruent both with your own healing and the healing of those with whom you share this world.

As in our own individual lives, healing on a global scale comes about as a function of our deepening awareness. It is one thing to take action that is informed by a rational, political, or ideological position—actions that are framed by "shoulds" and "shouldn'ts," which include rhetorical reasoning and, often, righteousness. It is another thing entirely to have such a deeply embodied sense of connection with the world that your actions are a natural representation of your commitment to living as a healing presence. Your life, then, is not operating out of ideology, but flow, and that flow has the natural quality of creating harmony everywhere it goes. In many ways, this is the deepest manifestation of what it means to be a healer. Your very existence is an invitation for others to step into a state of deep connection.

So, you start wherever you are with whatever you can. Every moment is the perfect moment to begin observing your experience without judgment, allowing curiosity to give way to wisdom, then allowing it to turn back into curiosity again. Hold on to nothing, treat yourself and others with kindness, and enjoy the ride.

Bibliography

Books that have had major impact to support me to LOVE MY BODY and TRANSFORM my HEALTH and HEALING:

Adyashanti, *The Impact of Awakening,* Open Gate Publishing, 2000
Adyashanti, *Emptiness Dancing,* Open Gate Publishing, 2004
Adyashanti, *True Meditation,* Open Gate Publishing, 2006
Adyashanti, *Falling into Grace,* Open Gate Publishing
Armstrong, Alison, **Keys to the Kingdom,** Pax Programs, 2003
Armstrong, Alison, **The Queen Code,** Pax Programs, 2012
Beckwith, Michael, **Spiritual Liberation,** Simon & Schuster, 2008
Berkson, D Lindsey, **Safe Hormones, Smart Women,** Create Space 2010
Bland, Jeffrey, **Your Health Under Siege,** Stephen Greene Press, 1981
Bland, Jeffrey, **Nutraerobics,** Harper & Row, 1985
Bohm, David, **The Essential David Bohm,** Routledge, 2002
Brown, Michael, **The Presence Process,** Namaste Publishing, 2005
Budd, Matthew, **You Are What You Say,** Crown Publishing, 2000

Castaneda, Carlos, *The Power of Silence,* Washington Sq Press, 1991

Chopra, Deepak, and Tanzi, Rudolph, *GOD: The Story of Revelation,* Harper One, 2012

Chopra, Deepak, *Super Brain,* Harmony Books, 2012

Ciaramicoli, Arthur, Kethcham, Katherine, *The Power of Empathy,* Penquin, 2001

A Course in Miracles, Foundation for Inner Peace, 1975

Coyle, Daniel, *The Talent Code,* Bantam Books, 2009

Csikszenthmihalyi, Michael, *Flow,* Harper Perennial, 1990

Dalai Lama, *The Transformed Mind - Reflections on Truth, Love and Happiness*, Holder and Stoughton, 2001

Dalai Lama, *Healing Emotions: Conversation with the Dalai Lama on Emotions and Health,* Shambala, 2003

Dalai Lama, *The Compassionate Life*, Wisdom, 2003

Das, Ram, *Be Love Now,* Harper One, 2010

Deida, David, *Intimate Communion,* Health Communications, 1995

Deida, David, *Blue Truth,* Sounds True, 2002

Deida, David, *The Way of the Superior Man,* Sounds True, 2006

Deida, David, *Dear Lover,* Sounds True, 2006

Dyer, Wayne, *The Power of Intention,* Hay House, 2006

Dyer, Wayne, *Wishes Fulfilled,* Hay House, 2012

Germer, Christopher, *The Mindful Path to Self-Compassion,* The Guilford Press, 2009

Hawkins, David, *The Eye of the I*, Hay House, 2001

Hawkins, David, *Power vs Force,* Hay House, 2002

Hopkins, Jeffrey, *Cultivating Compassion,* Broadway Books, 2001,

Levine, Barbara, *The Body Believes Every Word You Say,* Words Work Press, 2000

Lipton, Bruce, *The Biology of Belief, Mountain*, Love/Elite Books, 2005

Markides, Kyriacos C., *The Magus of Strovolos,* Arkana Penquin Books, 1985

McTaggert, Lynne, *The Field,* Harper Collins, 2003

Moore, Thomas, The Care of the Soul, Harper Collins, 1994

Nepo, Mark, *The Book of Awakening*, Conari Press, 2000

Osho, Love, *Freedom, and Aloneness,* St. Martin's Griffin, 2001

Paget, Lou, *How to Be a Great Lover,* Broadway Books, 1999

Pert, Candace, *Molecules of Emotion,* Simon & Schuster, 1997

Redfield, James, *The Celestine Prophecy,* Warner Books, 1997

Rosenberg, Marshall B., Nonviolent Communication, Puddled-ancer, Press, 2033

Roth, Geneen, *Women Food and God,* Scribner, 2010

Schwartz, Richard, *Internal Family Systems Therapy,* Guilford Press, 1997

Sheldrake, Rupert, *The Sense of Being Stared At,* Harmony, 2003

Sheldrake, Rupert, *New Science of Life,* Park St Press, 2009

Sheldrake, Rupert, *Dogs that Know When their Owners are Coming Home,* Three Rivers Press, 2011

Solomon, Robert, & Fernando Flores, Building Trust, Oxford Univ. Press, 2003

Singer, Blair, *The Little Voice Mastery,* XCEL Holdings, 2008

Talbot, Michael, The Holographic Universe, Harper Collins, 1991

Twyman, James F., *The Moses Code,* Hay House, 2008

Twist, Lynne, The Soul of Money, W. W. Norton & Company, 2003

Welwood, John, *Journey of the Heart,* Harper Perennial, 1990

Williams, Roger, *Biochemical Individuality,* McGraw Hill, 1998

Williamson, Marianne, A *Return to Love*, Harper Perennial, 1992

Williamson, Marianne, A Course in Weight Loss, Hay House, 2010

Whyte, David, *The House of Belonging,* Many Rivers Press, 1996

Young, Wm. Paul, *The Shack,* Windblown Media, 2007

Zaffron, Steve, & Logan, Dave, *The Three Laws of Performance,* Jossey-Bass, 2009

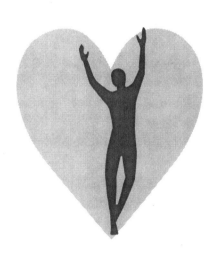

CPSIA information can be obtained at www.ICGtesting.com
Printed in the USA
BVOW01s0859200315

392564BV00004B/7/P

9 780989 648905